Quit smoking the easy way

How To Quit Smoking

A Happy Non-Smoker

Finlay J. Crawford

Quit smoking the easy way

Copyright © 2024 Finlay J. Crawford

All rights reserved. No part of this book may be reproduced or transmitted in any form or by any means, electronic or mechanical, including photocopying, recording, or by any information storage and retrieval system, without permission. in writing to the copyright owner.

ABOUT THE BOOK

This book is not just another quitting guide. It's a meticulously crafted roadmap that covers every aspect of quitting smoking, from understanding the deep-rooted causes of addiction to implementing effective coping strategies and long-term relapse prevention. Authored by someone who has walked the path and successfully quit smoking, this book shares a personal journey filled with insights, challenges, and triumphs. You'll find inspiration and motivation in the real-life success story woven throughout the chapters with a comprehensive quitting strategy. You'll discover why this method works and how it can be tailored to fit your unique needs.

What You Will Learn:
Learn to identify your personal, stress-related, and social triggers. Learn how to enlist the help of friends and family, seek professional assistance, and connect with online communities that share your goal.
Behavioral therapies like Cognitive-Behavioral Therapy (CBT), hypnotherapy, and mindfulness techniques. Learn how these methods can help rewire your brain and manage cravings.

Explore alternative quitting methods such as herbal remedies, acupuncture, and the role of exercise and nutrition in supporting your quitting journey.

Learn to recognize early warning signs of relapse, develop strategies to stay committed, and handle high-risk situations with confidence.

Benefit from contributions by health professionals and the latest research on smoking cessation. Gain expert insights that can enhance your quitting strategy. Reflect on your journey, embrace your smoke-free future, and receive final words of encouragement to help you stay the course.

Quitting smoking is one of the most significant decisions you can make for your health and well-being. **"How to Quit Smoking: A happy non-smoker"** provides the knowledge, tools, and support you need to make this life-changing transition. Empower yourself with the information and strategies in this book, and take the first step towards a healthier, happier, and smoke-free life today.

Table of Contents

CONTENTS

INTRODUCTION 8
   The Intent and Coverage 8
   My Journey And Success Story 9
Part I: Understanding Smoking 15
   The Psychology OF Smoking 15
   What Leads To The Habit Of Smoking? 18
      Who's Most At Risk Of Getting Hooked On Smoking? 18
      How Nicotine Affects You 19
   How Powerful Is Nicotine Addiction? 21
      The Challenge of Quitting Tobacco 25
   The Cycle Of Addiction: Exploring The Mental And Bodily Elements 27
   Common Myths About Smoking 30
   Health Threats and Results 38
      Cancers caused by smoking 41
   Immediate and Long-Term Health Effects 47
      The Impact of Secondhand Smoke on Those Around You 58
   Economic and Social Costs 66
      The Financial Burden of Smoking 66
      How Smoking Affects Your Social Life 69
Part II: Preparing To Quit 76
      Harnessing Visualization to Become Smoke-Free 92

Grasping What Sets Off Your Smoking	97
Navigating Social and Environmental Triggers	101
The Role of Friends and Family	104
Professional Help: Therapists and Support Groups	106
Online Communities and Resources	109
PART III: QUITTING METHODS	**113**
Cold Turkey: Is It Right for You?	113
The Pros and Cons	113
Success Stories and Tips	116
Gradual REDUCTIONS	121
Creating a Reduction Plan	121
Nicotine replacement therapy (NRT)	129
What's Next After NRT?	140
Behavioral Therapies	141
Cognitive-Behavioral Therapy (CBT)	142
How CBT Helps in Smoking Cessation	142
Structure of CBT Sessions	144
Hypnotherapy	145
How Hypnotherapy Helps in Smoking Cessation	145
Structure of Hypnotherapy Sessions	147
Mindfulness and Meditation Techniques	147
How Mindfulness and Meditation Help in Smoking Cessation	148
Practicing Mindfulness and Meditation	149
Alternative Approaches	151
Herbal Remedies and Natural Supplements	151

The Role of Exercise and Nutrition 156

Part IV: Staying Smoke-Free 160

    Managing Cravings and Withdrawal Symptoms 160

    Effective Coping Strategies 162

        Long-Term Withdrawal Management 163

    Staying Smoke-Free 166

        Spotting Early Red Flags 166

    Managing Tempting Times 174

    Cultivating a Health-Conscious Lifestyle 177

    The Significance of Nutrition and Physical Activity 182

        Embracing the Delights of a Non-Smoking Existence 186

Part V: Stories of Success and Inspiration 194

    Inspiring Stories of Quitting Smoking 194

        Insights from Their Experiences 200

    Expert Advice and Insights 207

        Latest Findings in Smoking Cessation 212

    Your New Beginning 220

        Words to Keep You Going 229

    Helpful Resources and Worksheets 233

    Progress Monitoring Charts 238

    Trigger Recognition Worksheets 242

    Commonly Asked Questions About Quitting Smoking 248

INTRODUCTION

THE INTENT AND COVERAGE

Think about smoking as a practice that goes beyond the individual, it ripples out, touching friends, family, and the wider community. The purpose of this guide is to equip you with the insights and tactics to kick the habit in a way that is both doable and sustainable. We're not just here to help you stop; we're here to make the journey as smooth and successful as possible. This guide is your ally, no matter if you're a long-time smoker who's faced setbacks in quitting or if you're just starting to notice smoking's toll on your health.

We've made sure this guide is thorough. It kicks off by exploring the mental and physical grips of smoking, shedding light on the 'whys' and the 'hows' of the addiction. With this knowledge, you can tackle the core issues head-on. Next up, we lay out a buffet of quit-smoking strategies, giving you the freedom to pick one that gels with your life and likes. And we don't stop there; the guide also sails into the waters of aftercare, arming you with the know-how to remain smoke free for the long haul.

Think of this guide as your quitting buddy, cheering you on and lending a hand throughout your entire quit-smoking voyage. It recognizes that quitting is a journey, not just a single leap, and gears you up for both the hurdles and the high-fives you'll encounter. By the time you turn the last page, you should feel pumped and ready to embrace a lifestyle free of smoke.

MY JOURNEY AND SUCCESS STORY

As for me, I began smoking at 18 because I wanted to be part of my peers and also believed it was a way of managing stress. What started as social smoking became my addiction. By the time I hit mid-twenties, I was consuming one pack in a day. Although, my attempt to stop turned out to fail every time. I struggled to manage my cravings.

A tipping point came when an ordinary checkup with my doctor who told me that there were signs of chronic obstructive pulmonary disease (COPD). The thought of living with any debilitating sickness scared me off completely. It dawned on me that it was not just about health but also the future and family commitment if quitting smoking is concerned.

Resolved to stop, I started searching for various ways and discovered that combining methods worked the best for me. I managed my physical cravings by applying nicotine replacement therapy while also undergoing cognitive-behavioral therapy (CBT). These CBT sessions enabled me to identify what sets me off and develop better responses. Additionally, I was able to locate a support group where I could exchange stories with others who were also in the process of quitting.

The prime lesson I learned was the need to have a good base of support. Among those whom I called upon included friends and family, seeking their advice about my discontinuing smoking decision as well as asking them to hold me throughout this walk. During moments when all seemed dim, their encouragement and sympathy were precious in many ways. In the same way, I changed my lifestyle by incorporating regular exercise and eating healthy diets. These adjustments also ensured that besides improving stress management levels in me, my overall well-being also improved greatly.

It wasn't easy. There were times when cravings got so strong that I just wanted to say "enough". But at each time, I reminded myself why I was quitting and what was waiting for me on the other side. With time however the craving gradually disappeared and I started enjoying plenty of benefits associated with smoke-free lifestyle. My health is miles better; no longer do I wake up spluttering with coughs, while having more energy and stamina than ever before. Additionally, there were substantial financial savings which could be channeled into more worthwhile experiences or investments.

Giving up smoking has been an incredibly difficult but fulfilling journey for me. It has taught me resilience, discipline, and the power of a supportive community. My success inspired me to write this book, with the hope that my story and the strategies I used can help others who are struggling with the same addiction. Quitting smoking is possible, and it is one of the best decisions you can make for your health and happiness.

You can join me as I explore more of my self-help journey also health, and fitness books, I will educate and share my expertise on with my fellow readers, as I see this as an opportunity to inspire and be your guide from the beginning to the end of the journey. More ways to get in touch will be included on my further work as this is my ever first book to write and get published. My weeks of work will surely give you the healthy life you seek. You can follow my Author Page for first hand info directly to your mail whenever I get a new book nor edition publish again.

Thank you and I appreciate you.

What Makes This Method Different?

There are numerous methods and resources available for quitting smoking, so what makes this book's approach stand out? The answer lies in its holistic, personalized, and practical approach.

1. **Holistic Approach**:

Many smoking cessation programs focus solely on either the physical or psychological aspects of addiction. This book, however, addresses both. It recognizes that smoking is not just a physical dependency but also a deeply ingrained psychological habit. By tackling both aspects simultaneously, this method provides a more comprehensive solution to quitting smoking.

2. **Personalized Strategies**:

Each smoker's journey is unique, and a one-size-fits-all approach is often ineffective. This book emphasizes the importance of personalizing your quitting strategy. It provides various methods, such as nicotine replacement therapy, gradual reduction plans, and behavioral therapies, allowing you to choose what works best for you. It also offers guidance on how to tailor these methods to fit your lifestyle, preferences, and specific triggers.

3. **Practical and Achievable**:

The strategies outlined in this book are designed to be practical and achievable, even for those with busy lives and limited resources. The book breaks down the quitting process into manageable steps, providing clear instructions and actionable tips. It focuses on making the journey as straightforward as possible, reducing the overwhelm that often accompanies smoking cessation.

4. **Support and Community**:

This method recognizes the critical role that support and community play in the quitting process. The book encourages you to seek support from friends, family, and professional resources. It also highlights the benefits of joining online communities and support groups where you can connect with others who are going through similar experiences. Sharing your journey with others can provide motivation, accountability, and valuable insights.

5. Inspiration and Real-Life Stories:

Throughout the book, you will find real-life success stories and testimonials from people who have successfully quit smoking using these methods. These stories serve to inspire and motivate, showing that it is possible to quit smoking, no matter how difficult it may seem. They also offer practical tips and insights from individuals who have been through the process themselves, making the advice more relatable and actionable.

PART I: UNDERSTANDING SMOKING

THE PSYCHOLOGY OF SMOKING

Smoking is a behavior shaped by a mix of mind-related, social, and body-related influences. Grasping what goes on in smokers' minds can steer us to craft better stop-smoking plans.

Psychological Factors

1. **Hooked on Nicotine**: Nicotine, tobacco's hook, tickles the brain into feeling good. Regular hits lead to a nicotine fix, sparking cravings, withdrawal fuss, and a smoking habit that's tough to shake off.
2. **Emotional Band-Aid**: For some, smoking is a crutch for the blues, nerves, or the dumps. While nicotine can briefly ease these feelings, smoking might just pile on more mental health woes down the road.
3. **Routines Run Deep**: Lighting up can turn into a hard-to-kick routine, with everyday stuff like hanging with smokers or certain moods flipping the smoking switch.

4. **The Reward Loop**: The quick fix smoking provides from stress or the comfort of the smoking ritual can lock in the habit, making quitting a tough nut to crack.

Social Factors

1. **Fitting In**: Puffing away can be tied to fitting in, especially in some friend circles. If your squad smokes, quitting can feel like climbing a mountain.
2. **Cultural Cues**: In some cultures, or groups, smoking's all the rage, making steering clear of smokes or the push to puff even harder.

Body Talk

1. **Genetic Hand**: Genes can nudge some towards nicotine's grip, especially if smoking runs in the family.
2. **Mental Health Links**: Those juggling mental health issues, like depression or anxiety, often light up more than others, maybe as a self-soothe tactic or because they're more in the path of smoking risks.

Quitting Game Plan

Kicking the habit usually calls for a mix of behavior change strategies, meds, and group support.

1. **Mind Shifts**: Behavior therapy can help smokers spot and swap out smoking triggers, learn stress-busters, and handle withdrawal woes.
2. **Med Help**: Meds like nicotine patches, varenicline (Chantix), and bupropion (Zyban) can be allies in the quit quest. Always chat with a doc to see what's best for you.
3. **Circle of Support**: Support groups offer a cheer squad, motivation, and buddies in the same boat, all rooting for a smoke-free life.

Getting why smokers smoke is key to creating quit-smoking tactics that truly work. By tackling the psychological, social, and biological roots of smoking, we can guide more folks to stub out the habit for a healthier life.

WHAT LEADS TO THE HABIT OF SMOKING?

A lot of smokers pick up the habit during their teenage years. It's more common to start if you're hanging out with friends or family who smoke. Some teens might light up out of curiosity or because it seems like a trendy thing to do.

Those flashy ads and promotions from the tobacco industry play a big role too. They pour billions into making smoking look fun, stylish, and harmless. Plus, we see smoking all over the place – in movies, TV shows, video games, and online. It's no surprise that studies link exposure to smoking on screen with a higher chance of teens trying it out.

Nowadays, e-cigarettes and other sleek vaping gadgets are also luring in young folks. They're often mistaken as a safe alternative and are super easy to get your hands on. These devices can be a stepping stone, teaching newbies how to inhale and getting them hooked on nicotine, paving the way to traditional smoking.

WHO'S MOST AT RISK OF GETTING HOOKED ON SMOKING?

Really, anyone who dabbles with tobacco could find themselves hooked on nicotine. Research points out that the teen years are prime time for this habit to stick. Start young, and your odds of battling nicotine addiction skyrocket.

The 2014 Surgeon General's Report tells us that nearly 9 in 10 smokers got their start before turning 18, and almost everyone who smokes started by 26. They also found that about 75% of high school smokers end up smoking into adulthood, even if they think they'll quit after a few years.

Is Smoking Truly Addictive?

Absolutely. Addiction means you keep craving and using something even though it's wreaking havoc on your life. It's like being emotionally chained to a substance. Nicotine, the culprit in tobacco, is super addictive – we're talking on par with drugs like heroin or cocaine. Regular tobacco use can quickly turn into a tough-to-kick addiction for many people.

HOW NICOTINE AFFECTS YOU

Nicotine, along with other substances found in tobacco smoke, gets quickly absorbed into your bloodstream through your lungs. Once it's in there, it spreads all over your body in a snap.

Now, in tiny doses, nicotine can actually make you feel pretty good. It helps you chill out and can take your mind off things that are bothering you. It messes with your brain and central nervous system, tweaking your mood. Nicotine's pretty sneaky—it hooks you by hitting your brain's reward buttons with a surge of dopamine, which is the same thing other addictive drugs do. Plus, it gives you a bit of an adrenaline boost. It's not a huge rush, but it's enough to get your heart going and your blood pressure up.

Here's the thing: once you take a puff, nicotine hits your brain in mere seconds, but the buzz fades fast, within a few minutes. Then you might start to feel a bit cranky and on edge. It's not like you're going through major withdrawal right away, but you get more and more uncomfortable as time passes. That's usually when you're tempted to light up again. When you do, the nasty feelings take a hike, and you're stuck in this loop. If you don't smoke again quickly, those withdrawal symptoms just keep getting nastier.

The more you use nicotine, the more your body gets used to it, and you end up using more tobacco to keep that nicotine buzz. This is what they call tolerance. Eventually, you hit a nicotine level that you're comfy with, and then you have to keep smoking just to maintain that level.

People who smoke can get hooked on nicotine super-fast, and kicking the habit can be tough. They can get all sorts of withdrawal symptoms like getting irritable, feeling jumpy, getting headaches, and having trouble sleeping. The real kicker is that even though they know smoking is wrecking their health and causing trouble with their families, they keep on doing it. That's addiction for you. Most smokers actually want to quit.

Scientists are digging into other chemicals in tobacco smoke that might make quitting an even bigger challenge. In animal studies, tobacco smoke seems to cause some brain changes that we can't pin down to just nicotine.

To give you an idea, a regular cigarette has about 1 to 2 milligrams of nicotine. But how much you actually take in can vary based on how you smoke, like how many puffs you take, how deeply you inhale, and other stuff like that.

HOW POWERFUL IS NICOTINE ADDICTION?

Nicotine addiction is incredibly strong. Roughly two-thirds of smokers express a desire to quit, and half of them actually make an attempt each year. Yet, only a handful find success without assistance. This struggle stems from a dual dependence on nicotine—both physical and emotional. Nicotine can influence a person's behavior, mood, and emotions significantly. For many, smoking becomes a way to cope with negative emotions, making it tough to give up. Smoking often becomes intertwined with social and other daily activities, further complicating the effort to quit.

Interestingly, kicking the smoking habit might be even more challenging than breaking free from drugs like cocaine or heroin. A 2012 review of 28 studies on addiction cessation revealed that while around 18% managed to stop drinking and over 40% succeeded in quitting opiates or cocaine, a mere 8% were successful in quitting smoking. This highlights just how formidable nicotine addiction can be.

Nicotine In Cigars

When it comes to cigars, those who inhale the smoke can absorb nicotine into their lungs as swiftly as cigarette smokers do. However, if you don't inhale, the nicotine absorption happens more leisurely through the mouth's lining. This means cigar smokers can still get their nicotine fix without having to breathe the smoke deep into their lungs.

Looking at the nicotine content, a typical full-size cigar packs a punch with as much nicotine as several cigarettes do. While a cigarette might have around 8 milligrams (mg) of nicotine, it actually delivers about 1 to 2 mg to the smoker. In contrast, many big-name cigars contain anywhere from 100 to 200 mg, with some even reaching up to 444 mg of nicotine. The amount of nicotine that ends up in a cigar smoker's system can vary widely, even among folks puffing on the identical brand. Factors influencing this include:

- The duration of smoking the cigar
- The number of puffs taken
- Whether the smoke is inhaled or not

Given these variables and the vast array of cigar sizes, pinning down the exact amount of nicotine delivered by larger cigars is pretty tricky.

Now, those little cigars that look and feel like cigarettes? They carry roughly the same nicotine content as a cigarette. If smoked in the same way as cigarettes (with inhalation), they're expected to provide a similar nicotine hit – that's 1 to 2 mg.

Nicotine In Smokeless Tobacco

Moving on to smokeless tobacco, this stuff really brings a hefty dose of nicotine. Once it's in your mouth or nose, nicotine hops into the bloodstream and travels to every corner of your body.

The nicotine content in smokeless tobacco is expressed in milligrams (mg) per gram (g) of tobacco, and boy, does it vary. We're talking about a range from 4 to 25 mg/g for moist snuff, 11 to 25 mg/g for dry snuff, and 3 to 40 mg/g for chewing tobacco. The amount of nicotine absorbed also depends on factors like:

- The brand of tobacco
- The product's pH level (its acidity)
- How much is chewed
- The cut of the tobacco

But at the end of the day, the nicotine levels in the blood of smokeless tobacco users are pretty much on par with those who smoke cigarettes.

Nicotine In Alternatives To Traditional Smoking

Various alternatives to traditional smoking exist, offering different methods of consuming nicotine without burning tobacco. These alternatives still carry the risk of nicotine dependence.

- Heat-not-burn cigarettes use a heating element to warm tobacco to a lower temperature than burning cigarettes, producing a vapor that users inhale.
- Edible forms of tobacco, such as lozenges, strips, gummies, or sticks, can be discreet and sometimes resemble sweets.
- Nicotine gels are products applied to and absorbed by the skin.

Nicotine in Vaping Devices

Vaping liquids in e-cigarettes usually contain nicotine, but the concentration can vary. Not all products accurately disclose their nicotine content.

Some e-cigarettes claim to be free of nicotine but have been found to contain it nonetheless.

THE CHALLENGE OF QUITTING TOBACCO

Quitting tobacco can be tough due to nicotine withdrawal, which affects you physically, mentally, and emotionally. Physically, your body misses the nicotine. Mentally, you're breaking a habit, which requires a significant behavioral shift. Emotionally, it might feel like losing a close friend. Quitting smokeless tobacco can be just as hard as stopping smoking.

Regular tobacco users will experience withdrawal if they suddenly cut down or quit. While withdrawal isn't dangerous, it can be quite uncomfortable, starting within hours and peaking around 2 to 3 days later as nicotine leaves the body. Withdrawal can last from several days to weeks, but symptoms lessen as one remains tobacco-free.

Withdrawal symptoms may include:

- Temporary dizziness
- Depression
- Feelings of frustration, impatience, and anger
- Anxiety
- Irritability
- Sleep disturbances
- Difficulty concentrating
- Restlessness or boredom
- Headaches
- Fatigue
- Increased appetite and potential weight gain
- Slower heart rate
- Digestive issues like constipation and gas
- Respiratory symptoms like cough, dry mouth, sore throat, and nasal drip
- Chest tightness

These symptoms can tempt someone to resume tobacco use to alleviate the discomfort.

THE CYCLE OF ADDICTION: EXPLORING THE MENTAL AND BODILY ELEMENTS

Addiction is a multifaceted illness that encompasses both the body and mind. While the bodily symptoms of withdrawal pose a significant barrier to quitting, they only represent part of the challenge. Psychological factors also play a crucial role, driving individuals with an opioid addiction into a potent cycle of addiction that unfolds in eight distinct phases.

What Constitutes the Eight Phases of The Mental Cycle of Addiction?

This cycle of addiction is marked by a series of thoughts and emotions, ranging from initial cravings to a loss of self-control, followed by pledges to stop, and eventually reverting to daydreaming about the drug. These patterns are intertwined with alterations in brain chemistry, further complicating efforts to cease drug use. Those grappling with opioid addiction may experience these phases several times daily or progress through them more gradually.

Here are the eight phases of the mental cycle of addiction:

1. Exasperation

Initially, individuals might turn to opioids in the hope of finding solace from persistent negative emotions like anxiety, fear, or depression. Opioids can provide a temporary escape by inducing euphoria, seemingly offering a way to mitigate these internal struggles.

2. Daydreaming

Before actual drug use, individuals might start to daydream about the sensation's opioids could provide and the relief they anticipate. They might also contemplate how to acquire a prescription or where to find opioids illegally.

3. Preoccupation

I can't stop thinking about using opioids right now. The belief that life would improve with substance use can lead to detailed planning regarding the timing and means of obtaining and using the drug.

4. Commencing Opioid Use

When overwhelmed by their thoughts and emotions, individuals may convince themselves that illicit substances will deliver the desired reprieve.

5. Spiraling Out of Control

Opioid addiction often results in a loss of control over usage, with individuals struggling to regulate the quantity or frequency of their drug intake.

6. Facing the Fallout

Addiction takes a toll on all areas of life, including personal relationships, employment, and finances. The resulting issues, such as broken relationships, legal troubles, and job loss, often provoke feelings of regret, guilt, or shame.

7. Halting Opioid Use

Reaching a crisis point, individuals may abruptly quit using opioids, vowing to themselves and others to steer clear of the substance for good.

8. The Lapse of Time

Despite the determination to stop, the appeal of addiction can be irresistible. As time passes, the initial discomfort that led to drug use resurfaces, and individuals find themselves back at square one, facing the same exasperation and daydreams that sparked their initial use.

COMMON MYTHS ABOUT SMOKING

Are you holding onto any misconceptions about smoking or kicking the habit? Let's take a closer look.

Nicotine addiction can cloud your judgment, making it hard to see the truth about tobacco and the quitting process. The tobacco industry's advertising and marketing can spread these myths, leading smokers to make excuses to keep lighting up. To quit successfully, it's crucial to challenge this "nicotine filter" and critically assess these myths. Here are a few more myths and the reasons they just don't hold up.

No matter your age, how long you've smoked, or what your gender is, the truth is that quitting smoking will boost your health. However, there's a lot of false information out there about giving up cigarettes, so let's debunk some of the widely held but incorrect beliefs.

MYTH: QUITTING IS POINTLESS NOW; THE HARM IS IRREVERSIBLE.

Even if you stop smoking later in life, say at 60, you could add three years to your lifespan compared to if you kept puffing away. Plus, a lot of the negative health impacts from smoking begin to reverse surprisingly quickly after you quit.

MYTH: NICOTINE IS THE NASTIEST THING IN CIGARETTES.

Sure, nicotine hooks you, but it's not the deadliest ingredient. Cigarettes pack over 7,000 harmful substances, including tar and carbon monoxide, not to mention 70 substances that could cause cancer.

MYTH: SMOKING WHILE ON NICOTINE REPLACEMENT THERAPY (NRT) IS A NO-GO.

Actually, research hasn't turned up any alarming side effects from using NRT while you smoke. Many folks on NRT are gradually smoking less, so they're taking in less nicotine overall.

MYTH: " SMOKING WON'T NEGATIVELY IMPACT MY HEALTH."

That's wishful thinking. The reality is that tobacco smoke doesn't discriminate. Half of all regular smokers will die from smoking-related causes, and the majority will face health problems and a lower quality of life due to their habit. Believing you're immune is simply not realistic.

MYTH: "SMOKING CHILLS ME OUT."

Not true. Smoking actually adds to stress. The moment the nicotine levels drop after finishing a cigarette, your brain starts craving another fix, making you feel edgy and stressed. While taking a drag might feel like stress relief, it's really just satisfying that craving.

MYTH: "SMOKING'S BAD, BUT SO ARE LOTS OF OTHER THINGS."

Smoking's impact is massive, causing thousands of deaths and untold health issues. It's a leading preventable cause of death, and its effects are far worse than many other health risks. Sure, life's unpredictable, but smoking is like walking into traffic without looking – it's a clear risk to your health.

MYTH: "I'LL PACK ON POUNDS IF I QUIT."

Most quitters don't gain significant weight, and those who do often shed the extra pounds over time. Plus, the healthy habits you develop when quitting smoking, like eating better and exercising, can help you maintain a healthy weight.

MYTH: "I'M YOUNG."

It's a common tale: young smokers often think they won't be puffing away in the future, but stats show many are still lighting up years later. Youth doesn't shield you from addiction, and nicotine's grip is tight. Don't fall for the myth that quitting will be easy later on. Now is the time to break the habit.

MYTH: "SMOKING IS A SYMBOL OF ALLURE."

That's just smoke and mirrors from the tobacco industry. In reality, smoking leads to wrinkles, yellow teeth, and bad breath—hardly the hallmarks of glamour. Plus, most folks find the smell of cigarettes off-putting. And let's not forget: smoking can dampen your love life and make you less appealing. Confidence and good health are the real attractive traits, not a cigarette in hand.

MYTH: "ONE CIGARETTE IS HARMLESS."

Have you ever heard the phrase 'One drag away from a pack a day"? It's a slippery slope. Just like you wouldn't tell someone recovering from other addictions to indulge 'just once,' the same goes for smoking. That one cigarette can reignite addiction and bring on feelings of guilt, leading to more smoking. The truth is, casual smokers often end up regulars or quit entirely.

MYTH: "I SMOKE 'LIGHT' OR JUST A BIT, SO IT'S NOT THAT BAD."

Don't be fooled. "Light" cigarettes pack the same toxic punch, and smoking even a little can harm your health. People often end up smoking more or inhaling deeper to satisfy cravings. And no matter how little you smoke, the risks to your health are still significant.

MYTH: "QUITTING SMOKING COLD TURKEY IS BEST."

Quitting smoking is a battle against addiction, and going cold turkey isn't always the answer. It takes a solid plan and the right mindset. Viewing quitting as a gift to yourself rather than a loss can make all the difference. While some succeed this way, it's usually with a lot of thought and a clear stance against smoking.

MYTH: "QUITTING SMOKING IS A BREEZE."

If only that were true. Nicotine is a tough addiction to beat, often rated more challenging to overcome than heroin or cocaine. Tobacco companies have engineered their products to be highly addictive. Quitting takes determination, planning, and a positive outlook.

MYTH: "I GENUINELY ENJOY SMOKING."

This is addiction talking. Just like any substance dependence, it's not about enjoyment; it's about not feeling lousy without it. Smoking becomes a crutch, and quitting feels daunting because of how integral it is to a smoker's routine.

MYTH: "SMOKING IS THE EPITOME OF COOL."

While smoking once had a reputation for being trendy, those days are long gone. Now, the side effects like bad breath, yellow teeth, and smelly clothes are seen for what they are—uncool. The image of smoking has taken a nosedive, and most people view it negatively.

MYTH: "MY SMOKING DOESN'T IMPACT ANYONE ELSE."

Think again. Second-hand smoke can harm others, causing serious health issues. Moreover, the tobacco industry often relies on child labor, and its environmental impact is significant, from deforestation to littering. Your smoking habit reaches further than you might think, affecting others and the planet.

MYTH: "SMOKING IS ONLY FATAL FOR THE ELDERLY."

While it's true that many smoking-related ailments show up after 50, the harsh reality is that smoking can cut lives short at any age. Even folks in their late 20s or early 30s can succumb to smoking-related diseases. These are not just brief illnesses; they're often chronic, excruciating, and can lead to an untimely death. But don't think you're off the hook if you're younger. Smoking can hit you with nasty conditions like gangrene, ulcers, and breathing issues way before you hit your golden years. The bottom line is, the sooner you start puffing away and the longer you do it, the higher your odds of falling ill because of it. Plus, smokers, regardless of age, tend to catch more colds, the flu, pneumonia—you name it—compared to folks who've never smoked or have kicked the habit.

MYTH: "I'LL JUST QUIT SMOKING WHEN I'M PREGNANT."

Thinking about having a baby? Well, smoking might throw a wrench in those plans since it's linked to infertility. And if you're lighting up while expecting, you're upping the risk of miscarriage and other pregnancy complications. Research is crystal clear: tobacco's nasty chemicals are no good for your baby's development. And if you smoke during pregnancy, your kid could face a bunch of health issues down the line. Quitting isn't a walk in the park—it often takes several tries. So, the sooner you start trying to ditch the habit, the better your chances of being smoke-free when you're ready for a little one. Despite good intentions, many women find it tough to stop smoking even when they've promised themselves, they would if they got pregnant.

HEALTH THREATS AND RESULTS

About 50% of all smokers die from smoking-related diseases.

It was calculated that there were approximately 5,950 deaths due to smoking in 2015; this figure is coupled with an estimated additional 100 fatalities resulting from secondary smoke. Furthermore, some 205,100 patients were admitted to hospital (including day case admissions and outpatient appointments) for conditions related to tobacco use or exposure to second-hand smoke.

The following are the statistics:

- Cancers – Half of them
- Circulatory diseases – Fourteen percent of them
- Respiratory diseases – Over half of them
- All causes – Thirty per cent of them.

Smoker's Health Risks

How does smoking damage your health? Check out the dangers associated with smoking.

Cancers

Smoking is by far the biggest single cause of lung cancer. It also plays a role in causing other types of cancer as well.

Heart disease

- Your heart is like the engine in your body. If you smoke,
- It makes your heart beat faster so that it requires more oxygen in your blood.

- Smoke will contain CO_2 gas which may produce blockages at heart arteries leading to people suffering from coronary artery disease or even experiencing heart attack.
- Smoking also increases a person's risk for blood clots.
- The arteries will become narrower, stiffer and less flexible thus reducing their elasticity and efficiency as they transport blood towards the heart.

Stroke

The risk of stroke (blood-clot, brain hemorrhage) is higher for smokers than non-smokers. It's one of the leading causes of death and long-term disability.

Bronchitis and emphysema

It can induce or aggravate these serious respiratory problems. Serious cases of emphysema cause breathlessness that may be worsened by infections.

Fertility levels and birth problems

Smoking tends to decrease fertility, while smoking during pregnancy leads to miscarriage, stillbirth and disease in infancy.

CANCERS CAUSED BY SMOKING

Lung cancer is primarily associated with smoking but it is also an established risk factor for different types of cancers.

In Ireland and many other countries cancer is a major reason for illness and death. If you are a smoker, your chances of getting any of the cancers listed below are greater (in some instances much greater).

Lung cancer

Almost half the population in Ireland would have been affected by lung cancer. In 2011, two thousand five hundred people developed lung cancer and 9 out of 10 were as a result from smoking.

It does not only affect smokers alone. The non-smokers who inhale smoke emitted by other persons or "second-hand" smoke have increased chances of suffering from lung tumors. There is a possibility that children and teenagers who breathe in second-hand smoke could develop lung cancer when they grow up. In addition, they might be at a heightened danger of getting asthma and other respiratory issues.

Mouth, head and neck cancer

Tobacco use is the leading cause of oral cavity (tongue, lips, gums) and mouth oropharyngeal cancer.

Cancer of the stomach

When you breathe in cigarette smoke, even if not on purpose you will always ingest some. The result is that smokers have an increased risk of developing stomach cancer.

Cancer of the pancreas

Smoking has been linked with pancreatic malignancy as it is considered a contributory factor if not causal.

Cancer of the kidney

In so far as kidney cancers are concerned too smoking has been identified as at least contributing to this disease development; although it may also be a causative agent.

Cancer of the womb (uterus)

It increases your chances for developing uterine cancer.

Cervical cancer

Female smokers have a higher chance of having cervical cancer than non-smokers do.

Cancer of the bladder

Smoking has been implicated in bladder carcinoma cases as well.

Cancer of the colon

Also known as bowel or rectal cancer, recent studies show that smoking cigarettes causes colon tumors.

Myeloid Leukaemia

A higher risk of developing myeloid leukaemia is associated with tobacco smokers.

The Health Effects of Smoking

Almost all parts of the body are damaged by smoking. Several diseases come from smoking and cause poor health among smokers generally.

- Smoking and Death
- Smoking kills people.
- Adverse health effects from cigarette smoking result in an estimated 443,000 deaths, or nearly one of every five deaths, each year in the United States.
- More people die annually due to tobacco use than those who die from HIV (Human Immunodeficiency Virus), illegal drug use, alcohol use, car accidents, suicides, and murders combined together.
- Men die due to lung cancer as a result of smoking at approximately 90% while for women it is estimated at about 80%.
- It is approximated that about 90% of total chronic obstructive lung disease mortality arises from cigarette smoke.

Smoking and Increased Health Risks

Cigarette smokers have been found to be two to four times more likely to develop:

- coronary heart disease
- stroke
- lung cancer in men (23 times)
- lung cancer in women (13 times)
- chronic obstructive lung diseases such as chronic bronchitis and emphysema (12-13 times)

Smoking and Cardiovascular Disease

Coronary Heart Disease is caused by smoking which has now become the leading cause of death in the United States.

Peripheral vascular disease, which is the obstruction of the arms and legs due to the obstruction of large arteries, from pain to gangrene is developed by smokers because smoking narrows the blood vessels (arteries) leading to reduced circulation.

Abdominal aortic aneurysm is a swelling or weakening of an artery in the abdomen and this happens due to smoking.

Cancer In Connection with Smoking

The following types of cancers have been associated with cigarette smoking:

- Acute myeloid leukemia
- Bladder cancer
- Cervix cancer
- Esophageal cancer
- Kidney cancer
- Larynx Cancer (voice box)
- Lung cancer
- Oral cavity (mouth) Cancer
- Pharynx Cancer (throat)
- Stomach cancer
- Uterine cancer

Smoking and other health effects Thus it can cause infertility; premature delivery; stillbirth; low birth weight; sudden infant death syndrome

(SIDS). For example, Bone density among post-menopausal smokers are lower than those who have never smoked.

Compared to women who did not smoke, women who used cigarettes exhibited more likelihood of hip fracture.

IMMEDIATE AND LONG-TERM HEALTH EFFECTS

The short- and long-term effects of smoking, explained

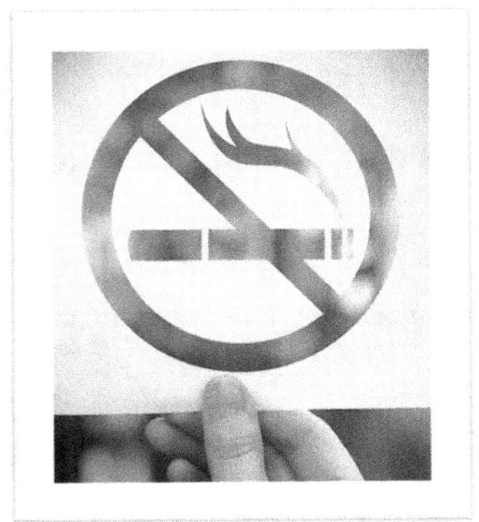

Smoking and its effects

There is no safe level of tobacco use. Every drug has different effects on individuals; for example, tobacco's impact may differ from one person to another depending on his or her physical characteristics such as size, weight and health and whether he/she has been used to taking it. Amongst other things, the effect of tobacco smoking differs from one person to another based on the quantity consumed.

In Australia, around 15,000 deaths are caused by cigarette smoking each year. In 2004–2005 about three quarter million hospital bed-days were due to tobacco use. (Collins & Lapsley, 2008)

It would be essential for anyone to ensure that appropriate care is taken when using any type of drugs.

What Are the Short-Term Effects of Smoking?

Tobacco smoking may therefore lead to:

- a general state of excitation followed by a decrease in activity within the cranial cavity
- increased vigilance and focus
- mild feelings of happiness
- sensation of relaxation

- increased blood pressure and heart rate
- reduced blood flow into fingers and toes
- cooler skin temperature
- halitosis
- suppression of appetite;
- dimness;
- discomfort in abdomen accompanied by nausea and vomiting,
- headache;
- coughing from smoke irritation.

Can someone die of nicotine overdose? Nicotine at very high doses can lead to an overdose. A 60 mg dose of nicotine taken by mouth is potentially lethal for an adult.

In other words, the person has consumed more nicotine than his or her body can handle. Some of the effects that come with excessive intake include:

- feeling dizzy
- bewilderment
- rapid reduction in both blood pressure and breathing frequency
- fits/convulsions
- a stoppage of breathing and death linked to hindrance of respiration.

What are some long-term effects of tobacco smoking? Smoking cigarettes causes tar to encrust their lungs, thus leading to lung and throat cancer. In addition, fingers and teeth among smokers are stained with yellow-brown coloration due to tar.

This CO combining with hemoglobin in cigarettes reduces amount of oxygen available for muscles, brain and blood. Therefore, it makes the whole body – primarily heart – work more difficultly. Over time this narrows airways and raises blood pressure which leads to heart attack or stroke.

At elevated levels they both boost the risk of cardiovascular disease, atherosclerosis and other circulatory disorders.

Some of the long-term problems that smoking may bring include:

- stroke and brain damage
- cataracts, loss of central vision, yellowing of the whites of your eyes (jaundice)
- no longer able to smell or taste things
- teeth stained yellow, tooth decay and bad breath
- nose cancer, lip cancer, tongue cancer and mouth cancer
- can cause you to go deaf.
- pharyngeal cancers and laryngeal are other effects.
- contributes to osteoporosis

- difficulty in breathing
- persistent coughing
- chronic bronchitis
- cancer
- triggered asthma attacks
- emphysema diseases
- heart diseases like heart attack or stroke,
- arteriosclerosis often leading to heart attack,
- high blood pressure (hypertension)
- myeloid leukemia which is a malignant disease affecting bone marrow and blood-forming organs.
- gastric bladder cancers and stomach cancers- ulcers occur here too.
- lower fertility rates, increased miscarriage risk,
- irregular periods/ cycles during menstrual cycle,
- decreased sexual desire in menopausal women.
- early wrinkles on face due to accelerated aging process though sunburns cause such marks too.
- slow healing wounds – I think this is a result of reduced cellular tension across cut sites hence less collagen production than usual creates such an environment for formation of wounds that take longer before they heal up completely.

- damaged blood vessels linings.
- susceptibility to increased infections
- damaged or low sperm production,

Other Consequences of Smoking

Involuntary smoking

Involuntary smoking takes place when a person who is not actively smoking breathes in the smoke from those people who are actively smoking. It irritates eyes and nose as well as causes such issues as heart disease and cancer of the lungs. Thus, it is particularly dangerous to infants and very young children.

Using tobacco along with other drugs

Nicotine can interfere with the way the body handles many different medicines. This can affect how these medications work. For instance, nicotine may make benzodiazepines less effective. Smoking while using birth control pills increases the risk that blood clots will form.

Ask your doctor or pharmacist if nicotine could potentially interact with any prescription or over-the-counter drugs you use.

Pregnancy and breastfeeding

   a. Many medications go through placenta into an unborn baby.
   b. Overall, perinatal drug usage may increase preterm delivered babies. This leads to low-birth-weight babies than usual.
   c. Drugs used by a mother during breastfeeding may be present in her milk – this could affect her baby's health too.
   d. Ask your healthcare provider before taking or considering taking any medications during pregnancy or while breast-feeding.

Tolerance and Dependence

If someone habitually consumes tobacco, he or she may become tolerant to nicotine. This implies that they require more tobacco smoking in order to achieve a similar effect.

They could easily get addicted to nicotine. It can be either psychological or physical addiction or both. Nicotine which is an addictive substance may become one of the most important things for an addict. Once they start using it, they cannot do without it since they have a strong desire for it.

Psychological dependence on nicotine makes one feel like smoking when he/she is in certain places or even with particular friends.

When the human body gets used to functioning while having nicotine present, this is known as physical dependency.

The Impact on Mental Health

For many years now there has been a debate as to whether or not smoking affects mental health. We are fortunate that we now understand through advances in technology and improved understanding of how the many different chemicals in smoke interact with the brain what harm smoking does to our mental health.

Utilizing smoking as a coping mechanism for mental health conditions may inadvertently inflict more damage on your physical well-being. Public Health England reports that individuals with mental health challenges account for one-third of cigarette consumption in England. Irrespective of mental health status, continued smoking raises the risk of health complications, making reduction or cessation vital.

Impact of Smoking on Mental Well-being

The interconnection between physical and mental health is profound. An impaired physical state can detrimentally affect mental well-being, often without immediate recognition. Research indicates a correlation between smoking, higher smoking rates, and increased risks of depression and schizophrenia. Cigarettes contain numerous toxic substances, including:

- Nicotine, which is highly addictive and leads to withdrawal symptoms.
- Carbon Monoxide, which hinders blood oxygen transport.
- Tar, a sticky substance causing arterial blockages and potential cancers.
- Benzene, associated with bone marrow damage and increased leukemia risk.
- Arsenic, heightening the risk of various cancers.

Over 5,000 toxic chemicals are released when a cigarette burns, with at least 70 identified as carcinogens. These toxins can exacerbate mental health issues. Furthermore, smoking has been linked to psychotic disorders, with nicotine adversely affecting the brain in ways similar to schizophrenia.

Nicotine's Role in Mental Health

Individuals with depression are twice as likely to smoke, and those with schizophrenia are thrice as likely. Nicotine's perceived benefits play a significant role in this relationship. Addiction to nicotine perpetuates the cycle of quitting and relapse, especially for those managing mental health symptoms.

Nicotine intake prompts the adrenal glands to release hormones like adrenaline and dopamine, offering temporary relief from mental health symptoms. However, unplanned cessation can lead to overwhelming withdrawal symptoms, prompting a return to smoking. While nicotine itself is not a major carcinogen, its withdrawal can be challenging and impact mental health.

Nicotine withdrawal symptoms include:

- Restlessness
- Irritability
- Headaches
- Fatigue
- Sleep difficulties
- Nausea
- Poor concentration
- Increased appetite

- Indecision

Psychological Benefits of Smoking Cessation

Committing to quitting smoking, with a structured plan, leads to improved physical and mental health. Benefits include reduced anxiety and depression, enhanced mood, a sense of well-being, increased energy, reduced stress, improved focus, and a boost in libido and appetite. The recovery process begins as early as 20 minutes after the last cigarette.

Support for Mental Health and Smoking Cessation

Quitting smoking can be challenging, particularly for those with mental health concerns. Support groups and advisors can provide assistance, while local pharmacies and GPs can offer connections to smoking cessation resources. Cognitive Behavioral Therapy (CBT) is also a valuable option, targeting the interplay between thoughts, behaviors, and emotions to break negative cycles.

Additional strategies include:

- Adopting a positive mindset
- Improving diet

- Engaging in physical activities
- Creating a cessation plan
- Keeping hands and mouth occupied
- Forming friendships with non-smokers
- Surrounding oneself with positive influences
- Using Nicotine Replacement Therapy (NRT) products
- Consulting a GP about medication options

Support is readily available for those struggling with smoking and mental health issues. With the right help and determination, quitting smoking is achievable.

THE IMPACT OF SECONDHAND SMOKE ON THOSE AROUND YOU

When you find yourself in proximity to tobacco smokers, such as during social events, you may unwittingly inhale secondhand smoke, also known as passive smoking. While immediate effects might not be noticeable, this exposure can have detrimental health consequences.

Understanding Secondhand Smoke

Secondhand smoke refers to the unintentional inhalation of smoke from burning tobacco products like cigarettes, cigars, or pipes. This smoke is a combination of the emissions from the lit end of the tobacco product and the exhaled smoke from the user. Non-smokers are not immune to the dangers posed by tobacco smoke. In the United States alone, secondhand smoke is responsible for thousands of deaths annually due to lung cancer and heart disease.

Alternate Terms for Secondhand Smoke Include:

- Passive smoking
- Environmental tobacco smoke (ETS)
- Involuntary smoking

The Dangers of Secondhand Smoke

Tobacco smoke from burning products is laden with harmful chemicals. Non-smokers breathing in secondhand smoke are exposed to these toxins, which can be more concentrated in the smoke from the unfiltered end of a cigarette, cigar, or pipe. Tobacco smoke contains over 7,000 chemicals, including approximately 69 carcinogens and 250 other harmful substances.

- ➤ Recognizable Toxic Chemicals in Tobacco Smoke:
- ➤ Benzene, found in gasoline
- ➤ Butane, used in lighter fluid
- ➤ Ammonia, present in cleaning products

- Toluene, an ingredient in paint thinner
- Cadmium, used in battery production
- Formaldehyde, used in fertilizers, embalming fluids, and building materials

Comparing Secondhand Smoke to Active Smoking

While active smoking is more hazardous to health, secondhand smoke exposure still poses significant risks due to the intake of harmful smoke chemicals.

Health Consequences of Secondhand Smoke

Both adults and children face serious health risks from secondhand smoke, including an elevated chance of lung cancer, heart disease, and respiratory infections.

Effects on Adults:

- Cardiovascular issues such as hypertension, arteriosclerosis, heart attacks, or strokes

- Respiratory conditions like COPD and asthma
- Increased likelihood of lung and breast cancer
- Reproductive issues, including low birth weight during pregnancy
- Regular exposure to secondhand smoke can increase the risk of heart disease by up to 30%.

Effects on Children:

- Increased frequency of coughing, sneezing, breathlessness, and other respiratory symptoms
- Recurrent ear infections
- More frequent and severe asthma episodes
- Respiratory infections like bronchitis or pneumonia
- Damage to eyesight and dental health
- Sudden Infant Death Syndrome (SIDS)
- Higher risk of brain tumors and lung cancer

To protect children and loved ones, it's advisable to cease smoking and seek guidance from healthcare professionals on the best cessation methods.

Duration of Secondhand Smoke Exposure

No level of secondhand smoke exposure is considered safe. Studies indicate immediate damage and inflammatory responses upon exposure, with significant effects occurring within minutes to hours.

Persistence of Secondhand Smoke in Enclosed Spaces

Secondhand smoke can remain in an environment for about five hours and may even spread through ventilation systems, posing risks to residents in multi-unit dwellings. Tobacco smoke particles can settle on surfaces and persist for months, known as thirdhand smoke.

Populations Most Vulnerable to Secondhand Smoke

Certain groups are more susceptible to the harmful effects of secondhand smoke:

- Workers in the service industry, such as restaurant and bar staff
- Infants, children, and pets, who may not have the option to leave smoke-filled areas

- Pregnant individuals, as secondhand smoke can reduce oxygen availability to the fetus, potentially leading to increased fetal heart rates, low birth weight, or premature birth.

Is it possible to develop cancer from inhaling secondhand smoke?

Indeed, inhaling secondhand smoke can lead to cancer. The Centers for Disease Control (CDC) reports that each year, over 7,300 non-smoking U.S. adults die from lung cancer linked to secondhand smoke exposure.

How can one minimize the risk of secondhand smoke exposure?

To reduce the risk of exposure, it is advisable to keep a distance from environments where smoking occurs. Refrain from frequenting places that permit smoking.

Although opening windows and using air filters may not eliminate all traces of secondhand smoke, they can contribute to reducing some of the harmful substances emitted from tobacco smoke. It is reasonable to request that people refrain from smoking in your personal spaces, such as your vehicle or home.

Additional measures to protect against secondhand smoke include:

- Seeking a smoke-free location if you encounter smoke.

- Choosing to visit establishments that enforce a smoking ban.

- Informing visitors that smoking is not allowed in your home.

- Prohibiting smoking in your vehicle, regardless of whether the windows are open.

Despite a decline in the number of tobacco smokers over the years, surveys indicate that around 25% of non-smokers are still exposed to secondhand smoke. The most effective strategy for protection is to maintain a distance from smoking individuals.

What is the prognosis for individuals exposed to secondhand smoke?

Continuous exposure to secondhand smoke can harm the heart and lungs. To maintain good health, it is crucial to steer clear of secondhand smoke. Fortunately, many municipalities and states have enacted public smoking bans in recognition of its health risks, though these do not entirely eliminate the risk of exposure.

When should one consult a healthcare professional?

If you find yourself frequently inhaling secondhand smoke, it may be time to discuss the associated risks and preventative measures with a healthcare professional. Should you experience heart or respiratory issues due to prolonged exposure to secondhand smoke, it is important to seek medical advice regarding treatment options.

Healthcare professionals may address specific symptoms or conditions resulting from secondhand smoke, potentially prescribing medication for high blood pressure or providing inhalers for asthma or COPD management.

A message from Finlay J. Crawford

While secondhand smoke may not be as detrimental as active smoking, it still poses significant health risks. Being aware of these risks enables you to safeguard your own health and that of others. Often, exposure to secondhand smoke occurs through contact with smokers. If someone close to you smokes, encourage them to quit for the benefit of everyone's health. Numerous resources are available to assist with smoking cessation.

ECONOMIC AND SOCIAL COSTS

THE FINANCIAL BURDEN OF SMOKING

Smoking is an expensive habit, one that extends far beyond the mere cost of purchasing cigarettes. The financial burden of smoking encompasses a wide range of direct and indirect costs, from the price of tobacco products to healthcare expenses and lost productivity. Understanding these costs can provide a powerful motivation for quitting, highlighting not only the personal health benefits but also the substantial financial gains.

Direct Costs

The most immediate and visible financial impact of smoking is the cost of purchasing cigarettes or other tobacco products. Depending on the region and the specific brand, a pack of cigarettes can range from a few dollars to over ten dollars. For a pack-a-day smoker, this quickly adds up to significant sums. For example, at an average price of $7 per pack, a smoker spends approximately $2,555 annually on cigarettes alone. Over the course of a decade, this amounts to over $25,000, a substantial sum that could otherwise be invested, saved, or spent on more meaningful pursuits.

Healthcare Expenses

Beyond the cost of cigarettes, smoking incurs significant healthcare expenses. Smokers are at a higher risk for a multitude of health issues, including lung cancer, heart disease, stroke, respiratory infections, and chronic obstructive pulmonary disease (COPD). These conditions often require extensive medical treatment, including doctor visits, medications, surgeries, and hospital stays. The financial burden of these medical expenses can be overwhelming, particularly in countries without universal healthcare. Even with insurance, the out-of-pocket costs for treating smoking-related illnesses can be substantial, encompassing deductibles, co-pays, and non-covered treatments.

Life Insurance Premiums

Smokers also face higher life insurance premiums compared to non-smokers. Insurance companies calculate premiums based on the risk of death and illness, and smokers are considered high-risk clients. This means that smokers pay significantly more for life insurance coverage. Over time, these increased premiums add up, further straining the smoker's financial resources.

Indirect Costs

Indirect costs of smoking include expenses related to property damage and maintenance. For instance, smoking can lead to fires, causing damage to homes, cars, and other personal property. Smokers may also face higher cleaning and maintenance costs, as smoke residue can stain walls, furniture, and clothing, and the smell can be difficult to remove.

Opportunity Costs

Finally, the concept of opportunity cost is crucial when considering the financial burden of smoking. Money spent on cigarettes is money that cannot be used for other purposes. By quitting smoking, individuals can redirect their funds toward more beneficial uses, such as saving for retirement, investing in education, traveling, or improving their quality of life in other ways.

HOW SMOKING AFFECTS YOUR SOCIAL LIFE

Smoking has far-reaching effects on social life, influencing relationships, social interactions, and overall social wellbeing. These effects can be both direct and indirect, shaping how smokers are perceived by others and how they navigate social environments.

Stigma and Social Perception

One of the most significant social impacts of smoking is the stigma associated with the habit. In many societies, smoking is increasingly viewed negatively due to its well-documented health risks and its impact on others through secondhand smoke. Smokers may be perceived as less health-conscious, less disciplined, or even less considerate of others' wellbeing. This stigma can lead to social isolation and decreased self-esteem, as smokers may feel judged or ostracized by non-smokers.

Relationships and Family Dynamics

Smoking can also strain personal relationships and family dynamics. Non-smoking partners, friends, or family members may express concern or frustration over the smoker's habit, leading to tension and conflict. The smell of smoke, the need for frequent smoking breaks, and the potential health risks posed by secondhand smoke can all contribute to relational stress. In some cases, this can lead to more serious issues, such as separation or estrangement, particularly if the smoker's habit is seen as prioritizing smoking over the wellbeing of loved ones.

Social Activities and Exclusion

The need to smoke can also limit participation in social activities. Many public places, such as restaurants, bars, and entertainment venues, have strict no-smoking policies. Smokers may find themselves stepping outside frequently to smoke, missing out on social interactions and feeling excluded from group activities. Over time, this can lead to a sense of isolation and decreased enjoyment of social events.

Impact on Children

For smokers with children, the social impact is even more pronounced. Children of smokers are more likely to experience respiratory problems, increased risk of smoking initiation, and the social stigma associated with having a parent who smokes. Additionally, parents who smoke may find themselves missing out on time with their children, as they step outside for smoking breaks or deal with smoking-related health issues.

Peer Influence and Pressure

Social circles can also influence smoking behavior. Smokers who spend time with other smokers may find it harder to quit due to peer pressure and the normalization of smoking within their group. Conversely, smokers who primarily associate with non-smokers may feel increased pressure to quit, which can be both a motivator and a source of stress.

Public Perception and Professional Relationships

In professional settings, smoking can affect career prospects and workplace relationships. Employers may view smoking as a sign of lower productivity and higher health risks, potentially influencing hiring and promotion decisions. Additionally, smoking can affect networking opportunities and professional relationships, as non-smoking colleagues may prefer to avoid smoke-filled environments.

Smoking in the Workplace

The presence of smoking in the workplace has significant implications for both employers and employees, affecting health, productivity, and workplace culture. Understanding these implications can help in creating policies and support systems that promote a healthier, more productive work environment.

Health Risks and Absenteeism

One of the most immediate impacts of smoking in the workplace is on health. Employees who smoke are at a higher risk for a range of illnesses, from respiratory infections to chronic diseases like heart disease and cancer. This increased risk translates into higher rates of absenteeism, as smokers are more likely to take sick leave. Frequent illnesses not only affect the smoker's health but also disrupt workflow and place additional strain on colleagues who may need to cover for absent employees.

Productivity Losses

Smoking also leads to productivity losses due to the time taken for smoking breaks. While a few minutes away from the desk might seem insignificant, these breaks add up over the course of a day, week, and year. For example, a smoker who takes four 10-minute breaks per day loses approximately 40 minutes of work time each day. Over a year, this amounts to over 160 hours of lost productivity per employee. For businesses, this translates into significant financial losses and reduced efficiency.

Workplace Environment and Safety

The presence of smoking in the workplace can also affect the overall environment and safety. Smoking indoors or in designated areas can lead to poor air quality, affecting both smokers and non-smokers. Secondhand smoke exposure is a serious health risk, linked to respiratory problems, cardiovascular disease, and other health issues. Ensuring a smoke-free workplace is essential for protecting the health and wellbeing of all employees.

Economic Costs to Employers

The economic costs to employers due to smoking are substantial. In addition to lost productivity and increased absenteeism, employers face higher healthcare costs. Companies often provide health insurance benefits, and the higher medical expenses associated with smoking-related illnesses can drive up premiums. This, in turn, increases the overall cost of providing health benefits to employees.

Legal and Regulatory Compliance

Employers must also navigate legal and regulatory compliance regarding smoking in the workplace. Many regions have implemented strict no-smoking laws in public and private workplaces to protect employees' health. Failure to comply with these regulations can result in fines and legal consequences. Employers need to ensure that their policies align with local laws and regulations to avoid these penalties.

Employee Morale and Retention

Workplace smoking policies can also impact employee morale and retention. Providing a supportive environment for employees who wish to quit smoking can improve overall morale and job satisfaction. Programs that offer smoking cessation support, such as counseling, nicotine replacement therapies, and wellness programs, demonstrate an employer's commitment to employee health and wellbeing. This support can enhance employee loyalty and reduce turnover rates, contributing to a more stable and positive workplace culture.

Social Dynamics and Inclusion

Creating a smoke-free workplace also addresses issues of social inclusion and dynamics. Non-smoking employees may feel more comfortable and valued in a smoke-free environment, leading to better teamwork and collaboration. Additionally, smokers who feel supported in their efforts to quit are more likely to engage positively with their colleagues, fostering a more cohesive and inclusive workplace culture.

Quitting smoking is a challenging but achievable goal, one that can lead to significant improvements in quality of life. By addressing the economic and social costs of smoking, this book aims to provide a comprehensive perspective on the benefits of quitting, empowering you to make informed and positive changes for your health and wellbeing.

PART II: PREPARING TO QUIT

Adopting the Correct Attitude

If you're determined to give up smoking, numerous strategies exist to help you maintain your commitment. We all aspire for this cessation attempt to be our final one and the one that endures for the rest of our lives. Our goal is to achieve lasting liberation from nicotine dependency as we extinguish that final cigarette and commence the healing process for our bodies. Formulating a strategy, exercising self-compassion, and maintaining an optimistic outlook are beneficial. It's equally crucial to look after your well-being, steer clear of other harmful habits, and adeptly handle your stress.

Overview

Fortunately, a variety of tips and techniques are available to assist you in breaking the smoking habit permanently. By understanding the dos and don'ts of quitting, as well as educating yourself about the effects of smoking cessation, you can increase your chances of successfully abandoning tobacco. Continue reading for valuable advice on how to quit smoking once and for all.

Essential Advice for Smoking Cessation

1. Develop a Strategy

Preparing in advance can ease your transition into the mindset required for smoking cessation and equip you with strategies to navigate the most challenging initial week to 10 days without cigarettes, as identified by the American Lung Association.

Schedule a health check-up and inform your healthcare provider of your intention to quit smoking. Discuss the most suitable options for nicotine replacement therapy or non-nicotine cessation aids for your situation.

Understand nicotine dependence.

Smoking transcends a mere "bad habit"—it's an addiction to a substance that alters your brain chemistry.

Set a "quit date." To maintain momentum, it's advisable to choose a date no more than a couple of weeks in the future.

Decide on your cessation method. You might opt for quitting "cold turkey" or prefer a gradual reduction approach.

Prepare for cravings. Compile a list of quick "craving busters" to distract from the urge to smoke, such as taking a walk, drinking water, solving puzzles, eating fruit, or calling a friend.

2. Consult Your Physician

Discuss your plans to quit smoking with your doctor. They can prescribe medications that may bolster your resolve to remain smoke-free.

Medications like Zyban (bupropion) and Chantix (varenicline) can be prescribed. Zyban may make nicotine less appealing, potentially diminishing the desire to smoke. Chantix aims to make smoking less satisfying.

Studies indicate both bupropion and varenicline are effective aids for quitting smoking, with varenicline showing a higher likelihood of continuous abstinence.

These medications have potential side effects, so it's important to discuss with your doctor which is best suited for you.

3. Explore Nicotine Replacement Therapies (NRT)

Products such as nicotine patches, lozenges, gum, and sprays can aid individuals in gradually reducing nicotine consumption, thereby alleviating withdrawal symptoms and cravings.

Research suggests that employing some form of NRT can enhance your probability of a successful quit by 50% to 60%.

NRTs are designed for short-term use, with a gradual decrease in dosage leading to eventual cessation.

4. Exercise Patience

It's natural to hope for a swift end to smoking cravings within a month. However, such expectations are often unrealistic.

Quitting smoking means overcoming an addiction that has likely been part of our lives for many years. It's reasonable to anticipate that breaking these longstanding associations and forming new, healthier habits will require time.

Consider smoking cessation a journey rather than a single event.

Take a moment to relax and view time as an ally in your quit journey. The more time that passes since your last cigarette, the stronger you will become. Maintain a state of patience with both yourself and the course of action.

Concentrate on the Present

In the early stages of smoking cessation, nicotine withdrawal can play tricks on your mind. The persistent thoughts of smoking can be overpowering, and the fear of not having cigarettes may trigger a return to old habits. When anxiety about a smoke-free future arises, refocus on the present day. It takes diligence and patience to remain in the present, but it is achievable and aids in managing your quit plan. Whenever your thoughts drift to the past or future, consciously bring yourself back by focusing on the present moment. Your ability to enact change is strongest today. Yesterday is past, and tomorrow is out of reach, but today is yours to shape.

Maintain a Positive Attitude Toward Your Achievements

It is often stated that a typical individual has around 66,000 thoughts each day, with a majority being negative, many of which we direct at ourselves. We tend to be our harshest judges. Remember, ceasing smoking is a journey, and a positive mindset can assist you through the inevitable highs and lows as you pursue your goals of quitting. Incorporate these strategies to keep a positive outlook in your cessation toolkit:

- Adopt affirmations for cessation. Choose several uplifting phrases to remind yourself of your strength and commitment, such as "I have the power to conquer nicotine," or "I prioritize my health above smoking."

- Maintain a journal of thankfulness. Keeping such a journal encourages a habit of appreciating life's positives and offers the benefits of stress relief through writing.

- Seek laughter. Finding humor, whether through a funny clip, a comedy show, or a humorous friend, can reduce stress and foster positivity.

- Practice self-compassion. Monitor your thoughts and eliminate any that are counterproductive, including regrets about unchangeable aspects of your past, like the time spent smoking.

- Celebrate the positive shifts. View previous attempts to quit not as failures, but as learning experiences that inform your current efforts to make positive life changes by quitting tobacco.

- Adopt "ignore mode" on difficult days. Acknowledge that bad days will occur. When they do, focus on distracting yourself from negative thoughts and moods.

- Rethink negative thoughts. When negative thoughts emerge, strive to replace them with positive ones, such as "I am making progress every day," or "This challenge is essential for my health."

Long-term cessation success begins with mindset

Prioritize Self-Care

During the initial phase of quitting smoking, it's crucial to pay extra attention to your physical needs. Tending to your body can ease the discomforts of nicotine withdrawal.

Here are tips to navigate withdrawal with greater comfort:

- Consume a balanced diet. Quality nutrition is vital as your body eliminates the toxins from cigarettes.

- Rest more. Fatigue is common during withdrawal, so allow yourself extra sleep. You'll likely feel refreshed and grateful for your smoke-free status upon waking.

- Hydrate with water. Water aids detoxification and can help curb cravings, contributing to overall well-being.

- Incorporate daily exercise. Physical activity improves both physical and mental health and is effective in managing smoking urges. It is important to seek advice from your doctor before starting a new exercise program.

- Take a multivitamin. Smoking depletes essential nutrients; a multivitamin can help restore energy levels during the first months of cessation.

- Although withdrawal is challenging, it's a temporary step toward recovery.

Limit Alcohol Consumption

Alcohol and tobacco are often used together, and studies indicate that individuals with alcohol use disorders have higher smoking relapse rates. Especially for new quitters, alcohol can be a trigger. It's advisable to avoid alcohol until you're more confident in your ability to resist smoking. Every person's journey to quitting nicotine is unique, so adjust your expectations accordingly.

If an upcoming event involves alcohol and causes concern, consider postponing your attendance until you feel stronger, or plan ahead for managing the event without smoking.

Quitting smoking is a life-saving endeavor that deserves your full commitment. Prioritize your cessation program for as long as necessary to maintain your smoke-free status.

Hint: My next book I will get published available on amazon would be on how to quit drinking. Anticipate!!!!!

Manage Stress Effectively

While addressing physical health is important during nicotine withdrawal, emotional well-being is equally crucial. Stress and anger are significant triggers for smoking and can jeopardize your cessation efforts if not managed properly.

Incorporate daily stress-relief practices to prevent becoming overwhelmed. Here are some activities to consider:

- Take a warm bath. A bath can be a serene escape that helps you unwind and forget about smoking.
- Go for a brisk walk. A quick walk can alleviate tension and stress.
- Practice visualization. Imagine a peaceful place to escape to when stress mounts.
- Enjoying personal time with a favorite book or hobby is not only pleasurable but also crucial for your quit program.

Seek Support

Statistics suggest that a robust support system increases the likelihood of long-term cessation success. Beyond friends and family, online support groups and forums can offer additional encouragement and resources.

Persevere

Many quit attempts are derailed by the thought that "just one" cigarette is manageable. Resist this notion; to overcome nicotine addiction, it's essential to avoid it entirely.

Stay Motivated

Keep in mind your reasons for quitting, and regularly revisit them to maintain clarity and motivation.

Quitting smoking is a process. Approach it one day at a time, and what once seemed arduous will transform into a rewarding challenge.

Cultivating the Will to Cease Unhealthy Habits

I was the person who frequently proclaimed, "I'm definitely going to quit smoking," using the declaration as a form of self-imposed accountability.

Yet, I harbored a secret certainty of my own failure, aware of my deeply entrenched habits. My vices were numerous: overeating, smoking, substance use, indulging in chocolate, excessive drinking, neglecting exercise, sloth, pornography, anger, depression, sorrow, lethargy, criticism, judgment, being overly opinionated, self-righteousness, and extravagant spending.

Many would flippantly advise me to "just quit," as if it were a trivial task—advice often dispensed by non-smokers. In retrospect, the act of quitting is straightforward, but why was it unattainable for me? Despite my efforts to educate myself through books and videos, I remained unable to master my impulses. I always questioned, "How exactly?" What worked for others seemed ineffective for me.

The Obstacle of Mindset

The crux of the issue lay in my mindset.

Even as I pen these words, feelings of inadequacy, another deeply rooted mental pattern, surge within me, clouding my thoughts and permeating my being with doubts about my authority, perfection, and credibility.

Despite these pervasive thoughts, I acknowledge my imperfections. I still occasionally drink, overeat, and smoke. I still harbor imperfect thoughts.

However, I've come to understand that these are all part of the journey towards "recovery."

Quitting smoking is ostensibly as simple as ceasing to smoke. Yet, I found it unattainable due to mental barriers. My cravings were triggered by anxiety, depression, anger, boredom, and even moments of happiness that falsely justified indulgence.

I recognized that my habits were interconnected, creating a web that ensnared me. Each habit reinforced the others, presenting a multitude of triggers that were overwhelming. Understanding this dynamic was one thing; overcoming it was another.

Developing a Strategy for Habit Transformation

I attempted various strategies with little success. What finally made a difference was the conscious removal of these habits from my mind, followed by the establishment of new ones. While the advice was to simply adopt new habits, I found that I couldn't until I had first eliminated the old ones.

Through meditation and reflection, I began to address each habit individually, discarding the associated thoughts, triggers, environments, and influences. Gradually, I managed to purge them from my consciousness.

This process was arduous and often felt insurmountable. Yet, with the aid of meditation, I have witnessed a transformation for which I am profoundly grateful.

The Evolution of Change

I am far from flawless, but I see progress. For instance, with exercise, I overcame the negative self-talk that once hindered me by surrendering those thoughts to a higher power. I ceased to engage with them and instead released them. This allowed me to establish new, positive habits.

Today, exercise has become integral to my life, and its absence is palpable. Thanks to meditation, I have managed to create a fertile mental ground for cultivating new patterns of behavior.

Currently, I am in the best shape of my life, with improved finances, health, mental stability, positivity, happiness, and self-control. The journey continues, but I am committed to moving forward.

Final Thoughts

In summary, the formula for changing habits is a function of the number and intensity of the habits, which together determine the difficulty of altering them. The initial step is to eliminate these habits from your mind, and then, on a clean slate, to develop new ones.

I hope my insights prove beneficial. If you require assistance, please know that help is available.

Setting Realistic Goals

Establish Objectives and Embrace a Smoke-Free Existence

Acknowledging your desire to cease smoking is a commendable first step. To enhance your likelihood of success, it's crucial to articulate your intentions clearly by setting a target date and objectives for quitting. Develop a strategy for the changes you wish to implement and consider how to maintain these changes over time.

Consider this a phased approach:

1. Reflect on your motivation for change – understanding why quitting is significant to you will bolster your commitment to your goal.

2. Define your objectives – pinpoint exactly what you're striving to achieve.

3. Devise your action plan – outline the steps necessary to accomplish your goal.

If the prospect of change feels overwhelming, break it down into manageable increments. Small victories can bolster your confidence and motivation. Even if these increments seem minor, they collectively steer you toward your ultimate goal. As you attain each smaller target or mini-goal, set new, more challenging ones to continue your progress.

We've designed a tool to assist you in setting a quit date, establishing goals, and outlining the incremental steps to take. Set a quit date, define your goal, and formulate action plans. If you prefer to set goals independently, a downloadable PDF version of the action plan is available.

Guidelines for Goal-Setting:

When formulating any goal, consider applying the SMART criteria:

- Specific – add details to clarify what needs to be done.

- Measurable – incorporate quantifiable metrics.

- Action-focused – ensure the goal pertains to a specific behavior.

- Realistic – select achievable goals.

- Timed – set a deadline for accomplishing your goal.

For instance, transform the goal "Remove all smoking-related paraphernalia from my residence" into a SMART goal: "Within the next two weeks, preceding my quit date of June 13, I will meticulously inspect each room of my house and discard any ashtrays, lighters, or other smoking-related items."

HARNESSING VISUALIZATION TO BECOME SMOKE-FREE

The Impact of Visualization on Smoking Cessation

Have you considered the influence your mind wields in your quest to quit smoking? Visualization, the process of forming mental imagery, can be an instrumental technique in conquering addiction. Mastering visualization to quit smoking can address the psychological and emotional hurdles associated with this endeavor. Let's delve into how this potent strategy can support your transition to a smoke-free lifestyle and enhance other cessation aids such as Smotect Natural Tablets.

Understanding Visualization's Significance

Visualization transcends mere daydreaming; it's an intentional practice where you envision yourself achieving a precise objective—becoming smoke-free, in this context. It's a strategy employed by athletes, business figures, and achievers globally. By harnessing visualization to quit smoking, you access a formidable mental asset that can solidify your dedication and elevate your confidence to surmount addiction.

Visualization Techniques for Smoking Cessation

Craft a Vivid Mental Picture:

Find a serene environment free from interruptions. Shut your eyes and conjure up a scenario where you successfully resist a smoking urge.

Envision the environment, the people present, and, most importantly, the sensations of self-respect and triumph.

Daily Visualization Practice:

Consistency is vital. Allocate time each day to imagine your life without smoking. The more regularly you practice, the more ingrained and realistic the visualization becomes.

Engage All Senses:

Enhance the vividness of your visualization by engaging all senses. What visuals, sounds, scents, and tactile sensations do you experience? The richer the details, the more impactful the visualization.

Positive Reinforcement:

Utilize visualization to affirm positive affirmations. Envision the advantages of not smoking, such as improved health, increased vitality, and a newfound sense of liberation.

Anticipate Challenges:

Employ this method to mentally rehearse confronting cravings. How will you decline a cigarette? Visualize navigating these situations with poise and assurance.

Advantages of Visualization in Smoking Cessation

Alleviates Stress and Anxiety:

Visualization can serve as a soothing exercise, diminishing the stress and anxiety linked to quitting.

Boosts Motivation and Confidence:

Regular visualization fortifies your resolve and enhances your self-assurance in your ability to quit.

Prepares for Actual Situations:

Mental rehearsal of challenging encounters better equips you to handle them in reality.

Enhancing Visualization with Smotect Natural Tablets

While visualization is a potent mental practice, pairing it with physical aids can render your cessation journey more efficacious. Smotect Natural Tablets, featuring a unique blend of 12 therapeutic herbs, aim to minimize cravings and repair smoking-induced damage. These tablets are 100% natural, non-addictive, clinically validated, FDA-approved, and GMP-certified. Incorporating these tablets into your regimen can offer physical reinforcement to the mental resilience built through visualization techniques.

A Comprehensive Approach to Smoking Cessation

Quitting smoking encompasses both physical and mental challenges. Learning to visualize smoking cessation equips you with a robust mental tool that, when combined with practical physical aids like Smotect Natural Tablets, presents a comprehensive strategy for overcoming addiction. Embrace the strength of your mind, bolster it with appropriate support, and confidently step into a smoke-free existence.

Bear in mind, each act of visualization propels you closer to your objective. With every mental depiction of success, you pave the path toward a healthier, more content, and smoke-free future.

GRASPING WHAT SETS OFF YOUR SMOKING

SPOTTING WHAT SPARKS YOUR CRAVINGS

A key element in ditching cigarettes is to grasp what kicks off your need to light up. These sparks, or triggers, differ from one person to another and are often rooted in our daily habits, emotional reactions, and social life. Spotting your own set of triggers is the foundational move to cut through the addiction loop.

Jotting Down a Smoke Log

To pinpoint your smoking triggers, try jotting down a smoke log. Over a couple of weeks, scribble down every instance you reach for a cig. Keep track of the time, your emotional state, your actions, and any extra details. This log will reveal patterns and spotlight specific scenarios or feelings that make you want to smoke.

You might notice you're puffing away more when you sip your morning coffee, after chowing down a meal, during work breaks, or whenever you're feeling tense or just plain bored. Recognizing these habits helps you get a handle on when those cravings tend to hit.

Routines and Their Role

Your day-to-day schedule has a hefty impact on your smoking habits. It's common to find that certain daily moments are tightly knotted with reaching for a cigarette. Maybe it's that automatic smoke with your morning alarm, during your drive, or when you're kicking back in the evening. These habitual triggers are tough nuts to crack since they're so routine.

The Emotional Angle

Feelings are big-time triggers, too. Lots of folks' smoke as a way to deal with the tough stuff—stress, worry, sadness, or just feeling empty. On the flip side, good vibes like joy or excitement can also lead to a smoke, as people use cigarettes to boost or celebrate a moment. Getting wise to these emotional triggers is a step toward swapping out smoking with healthier ways to handle your emotions.

The Social Scene

Hanging out in social settings can be a minefield for smokers. Being around others who smoke, going to events, or doing things where smoking is common can crank up the temptation. Wanting to blend in, especially if your crew or relatives are smokers, can also make it hard to resist.

Stress and Its Ties to Smoking

Stress and emotional responses are tricky when you're trying to quit. Smoking is often a go-to for managing stress, nerves, and other downer emotions. Figuring out how these emotional triggers tick and finding other ways to tackle stress is key for kicking the habit for good.

The Vicious Stress-Smoke Loop

Smoking can trap you in a nasty stress-dependence spin. Nicotine might seem soothing at first, but it actually jacks up stress over time. The irritability, jitteriness, and scatterbrained feeling that come with nicotine withdrawal can pump up stress, making smoking feel like both the problem and the solution.

Zeroing in on Stress Triggers

To snap the stress-smoke loop, work out what stress factors make you want to smoke. It could be job pressure, money woes, rocky relationships, or daily hassles like gridlock or looming deadlines. By calling out these stress triggers, you can start crafting ways to handle them without reaching for a smoke.

Crafting Healthier Stress Busters

After you've nailed down your stress triggers, it's time to build some healthier stress busters. Exercise is a top-notch stress reliever. Getting active pumps out endorphins, lifting your mood and cutting down on stress. A quick walk can have amazing effects.

Mindfulness and chill-out tactics, like meditation, deep breathing, and yoga, can also help you keep stress at bay. These practices foster relaxation and can curb the smoking urge by keeping you calm and collected.

Picking up hobbies or activities that chill you out is another solid move. Whether it's getting lost in a book, digging in the garden, painting, or jamming on an instrument, finding a positive way to channel your stress can drop your need to smoke.

Reaching Out for Support

Don't underestimate the boost you can get from friends, family, or pros. Sharing your struggles can lighten the load and offer fresh viewpoints. Support groups, whether face-to-face or online, can give you a sense of belonging and understanding that's super helpful when you're up against stress and the itch to light up.

NAVIGATING SOCIAL AND ENVIRONMENTAL TRIGGERS

Social and environmental triggers are those outside nudges that spark your smoking urge. They're often tied to places, activities, or social moments and can be a real challenge when you're trying to quit.

Tweaking Your Surroundings

A solid first step in dealing with environmental triggers is to craft a smoke-free zone. Toss out all your smoking gear from your place, car, and work area. Give everything a good scrub to get rid of that smoky smell, which can be a big trigger.

It's smart to steer clear of spots where you used to smoke, especially when you're fresh into quitting. If certain places or routines are closely linked to smoking, think about shaking up your schedule or finding new, smoke-free spots to hang out.

Social Triggers and How to Handle Them

Social triggers are all about the people you're with, especially if they're smokers. Being around smokers, whether they're buddies, family, or coworkers, can make it tough to say no to a cigarette. Social spots like parties, bars, or get-togethers can also tempt you to smoke, especially if they're part of your past smoking life.

Spreading the Word

A smart tactic for handling social triggers is to let your circle know you're quitting. Tell your pals, relatives, and workmates about your plan to ditch cigarettes and ask for their backup. They can help by not smoking around you and by getting why you might need to duck out of trigger-heavy spots.

Surrounding Yourself with Support

Finding a supportive crew can make a huge difference. Chilling with non-smokers or folks who are also trying to quit can rub off on you in a good way and lessen the urge to smoke. Support groups, both in person and online, can give you that sense of togetherness and understanding that's gold when you're trying to quit.

Forging New Social Routines

Creating new social routines that don't revolve around smoking can help you navigate social triggers. Look for activities and gatherings where smoking isn't the main event. Dive into hobbies, sports, or other interests that encourage a smoke-free way of life.

Getting Tough Against Triggers

Building up your defense against social and environmental triggers takes time. Each time you face a trigger and don't smoke, you're beefing up your resistance for the next time. Give yourself a pat on the back for these wins and recognize the strides you're making toward a smoke-free existence.

Building a Support System

The Role of Friends and Family

One of the most important factors in successfully quitting smoking is having a strong support system. Friends and family play a crucial role in this process, providing emotional support, encouragement, and practical assistance. Their involvement can make the difference between success and failure, as they can help you navigate the challenges and setbacks that are an inevitable part of quitting.

Open Communication

The first step in leveraging the support of friends and family is to communicate openly about your decision to quit smoking. Let them know why you are quitting, what your goals are, and how they can help. Explain the importance of their support and ask for their understanding and patience. By being open about your journey, you create an environment where they can provide the encouragement and assistance you need.

Emotional Support

Emotional support from loved ones can be invaluable during the quitting process. Quitting smoking is a significant lifestyle change, and having someone to talk to can help you manage the emotional ups and downs. Friends and family can offer a listening ear, provide reassurance, and remind you of your progress and reasons for quitting. This emotional backing can boost your morale and strengthen your resolve.

Positive Reinforcement

Positive reinforcement is a powerful motivator. Encourage your friends and family to acknowledge your efforts and celebrate your milestones. This could be as simple as offering words of praise, or it could involve more tangible rewards, like treating you to a special outing or gift when you reach a significant milestone. Positive reinforcement helps to build your confidence and reinforces your commitment to quitting.

Understanding and Patience

It's important for friends and family to understand that quitting smoking is a challenging process that may involve setbacks. Encourage them to be patient and supportive, even if you experience relapses. Rather than criticizing or expressing frustration, they should focus on encouraging you to keep trying and reminding you that each attempt brings you closer to success.

PROFESSIONAL HELP: THERAPISTS AND SUPPORT GROUPS

While support from friends and family is essential, professional help can provide additional, specialized assistance that can significantly enhance your chances of quitting smoking. Therapists and support groups offer expert guidance, structured programs, and a supportive community that can address both the psychological and physical aspects of addiction.

Therapists and Counselors

Therapists and counselors who specialize in smoking cessation can provide personalized support tailored to your specific needs and challenges. Cognitive-behavioral therapy (CBT) is one of the most effective approaches, helping you to identify and change the thought patterns and behaviors that contribute to your smoking habit. Therapists can also teach you coping strategies for managing stress and cravings, and they can help you develop a comprehensive quit plan.

Individualized Attention

One of the main advantages of working with a therapist is the individualized attention you receive. Therapists can help you explore the underlying reasons for your smoking, such as emotional triggers or stressors, and develop strategies to address these issues. This personalized approach can be particularly beneficial if you have tried to quit before and struggled with specific challenges.

Support Groups

Structured Programs

Many support groups follow structured programs that provide a step-by-step approach to quitting smoking. These programs often include educational sessions about the health risks of smoking, strategies for coping with cravings, and techniques for preventing relapse. The structure and accountability provided by these programs can help you stay on track and maintain your commitment to quitting.

Healthcare Providers

In addition to therapists and support groups, healthcare providers such as doctors, nurses, and pharmacists can offer valuable support. They can provide information about nicotine replacement therapy (NRT), prescription medications, and other treatments that can help reduce withdrawal symptoms and cravings. Regular check-ins with a healthcare provider can also help you monitor your progress and address any concerns that arise during your quitting journey.

ONLINE COMMUNITIES AND RESOURCES

In today's digital age, online communities and resources have become an increasingly valuable tool for individuals looking to quit smoking. These platforms offer a wealth of information, support, and tools that can complement traditional methods of quitting. They provide access to a broader community of people who are also trying to quit, as well as experts who can offer advice and encouragement.

Online Support Groups

Online support groups function similarly to in-person support groups, providing a space where individuals can share their experiences, challenges, and successes. These groups are accessible 24/7, allowing you to connect with others at any time of day. This constant availability can be particularly helpful during moments of intense cravings or stress.

Forums and Discussion Boards

Forums and discussion boards are another valuable resource, offering a platform for asking questions, sharing tips, and receiving feedback from a diverse community. These boards often have sections dedicated to different stages of the quitting process, allowing you to find relevant information and connect with others who are at the same stage as you.

Moderated forums can also ensure that the advice and information shared are accurate and supportive.

Mobile Apps

There are numerous mobile apps designed to help individuals quit smoking. These apps often include features such as progress tracking, goal setting, and reminders. They can also provide educational resources, tips for managing cravings, and daily motivational messages.

Educational Websites and Resources

Educational websites dedicated to smoking cessation provide a wealth of information about the health risks of smoking, the benefits of quitting, and strategies for success. These sites often include interactive tools, such as cost calculators that show how much money you can save by quitting, and quizzes that help you assess your readiness to quit. Many of these resources are created by reputable health organizations, ensuring that the information is accurate and up-to-date.

Social Media Communities

Social media platforms like Facebook, Reddit, and Twitter host numerous groups and communities focused on quitting smoking. These communities provide a space for sharing stories, asking questions, and receiving support from a diverse and global network. The interactive nature of social media allows for real-time communication and the sharing of multimedia content, such as videos and infographics, that can enhance your understanding and motivation.

Online Counseling and Coaching

For those who prefer professional support, online counseling and coaching services offer the convenience of accessing help from the comfort of your home. These services can connect you with trained counselors and coaches who can provide personalized guidance and support through video calls, chat, or email. This flexibility makes it easier to incorporate professional help into your quitting plan, regardless of your schedule or location.

Quitting smoking is a challenging process, but with the right support system in place, you can navigate the ups and downs with confidence.

Whether it's through the encouragement of loved ones, the expertise of professionals, or the connectivity of online communities, each element of your support system plays a crucial role in helping you achieve your goal of a smoke-free life.

PART III: QUITTING METHODS

COLD TURKEY: IS IT RIGHT FOR YOU?

The Pros and Cons

Quitting smoking "cold turkey" refers to stopping all at once, without the aid of nicotine replacement therapy (NRT), medications, or gradual reduction. While it can be an effective method for some, it comes with its own set of pros and cons. Understanding these can help you determine if going cold turkey is the right approach for you.

Pros of Quitting Cold Turkey

1. **Immediate Health Benefits**: Quitting smoking cold turkey means you stop ingesting harmful substances immediately, allowing your body to begin the healing process right away. Within just 20 minutes of your last cigarette, your heart rate drops, and within 12 hours, carbon monoxide

levels in your blood return to normal. These immediate health benefits can be a powerful motivator.

2. **Simplicity**: The cold turkey method is straightforward. There are no plans to follow, medications to take, or devices to use. This simplicity can be appealing, especially for those who prefer a no-nonsense approach.

3. **Cost-Effective:** Quitting cold turkey does not require purchasing NRT products or medications, making it a cost-effective option. This can be particularly beneficial for individuals who are motivated by saving money.

4. **Psychological Benefits**: For some, the all-or-nothing approach of quitting cold turkey can be empowering. Successfully quitting this way can boost your confidence and reinforce your determination to stay smoke-free.

5. **Shorter Withdrawal Period:** Although withdrawal symptoms can be intense, they typically peak within the first week and begin to subside after that. This shorter, albeit more intense, withdrawal period can be seen as an advantage over methods that involve a prolonged tapering process.

Cons of Quitting Cold Turkey

1. **Intense Withdrawal Symptoms**: The abrupt cessation of nicotine can lead to severe withdrawal symptoms, including irritability, anxiety, depression, headaches, and intense cravings. These symptoms can be overwhelming and challenging to manage without support.

2. **Lower Success Rates**: Statistically, the cold turkey method has lower success rates compared to methods that include NRT or medications. Many smokers find it difficult to cope with withdrawal symptoms and relapse as a result.

3. **Lack of Support**: Without the aid of NRT, medications, or a structured plan, individuals quitting cold turkey may lack the support and tools needed to manage cravings and withdrawal symptoms effectively.

4. **Increased Stress**: The stress of dealing with withdrawal symptoms can be exacerbated by external factors such as work, family, and social obligations. Stress without a support system can result in relapse.

5. **Potential for Relapse**: The intensity of withdrawal symptoms and cravings can increase the likelihood of relapse, especially if you don't have a solid plan for managing these challenges.

SUCCESS STORIES AND TIPS

Despite the challenges, many people have successfully quit smoking cold turkey. Their stories and tips can provide valuable insights and inspiration for those considering this method.

Success Story 1: Emily's Determination

Emily had been a smoker for over 15 years and had tried various methods to quit, including nicotine patches and gum, without success. Frustrated with her lack of progress, she decided to quit cold turkey. Emily set a quit date and prepared herself mentally for the challenge ahead.

She found that keeping busy was key to managing her cravings. Emily took up running and joined a local gym, using exercise as a way to distract herself and relieve stress. She also kept a journal to track her progress and reflect on her journey. When cravings hit, she reminded herself of the reasons she wanted to quit: her health, her family, and her desire for a smoke-free life.

Emily's Tips:

1. **Stay Active**: Physical activity can help manage cravings and reduce stress. Discover a physical activity that you love and incorporate it into your daily schedule.

2. **Journal Your Journey**: Keeping a journal can help you track your progress, identify triggers, and stay motivated.

3. **Remind Yourself of Your Reasons**: Write down the reasons you want to quit and refer to them when cravings strike. This can help reinforce your commitment to staying smoke-free.

Success Story 2: John's Support Network

John had been smoking for over 20 years and had developed significant health issues as a result. His doctor strongly recommended quitting, and John decided to go cold turkey. Recognizing the challenges ahead, he reached out to friends and family for support.

John's wife and children were incredibly supportive, helping him avoid triggers and providing encouragement. He also joined an online support group for people quitting smoking, where he could share his experiences and get advice from others going through the same process. Whenever cravings hit, John found solace in the support of his loved ones and the online community.

John's Tips:

1. **Build a Support Network**: Having a strong support system can make a significant difference. Reach out to friends, family, and online communities for encouragement and advice.

2. **Avoid Triggers**: Identify situations, places, and activities that trigger your urge to smoke and try to avoid them, especially in the early stages of quitting.

3. **Stay Positive**: Focus on the benefits of quitting and celebrate your progress. Your confidence and motivation can be enhanced through positive reinforcement.

Success Story 3: Sarah's Mindfulness Practice

Sarah had attempted to quit smoking multiple times using various methods but always ended up relapsing. Determined to make a lasting change, she decided to quit cold turkey and incorporate mindfulness practices into her routine.

Sarah began practicing meditation and deep breathing exercises daily, which helped her manage stress and cravings. She also attended mindfulness workshops and read books on the subject to deepen her understanding. By staying present and focusing on her breath, Sarah found it easier to navigate the challenges of quitting.

Sarah's Tips:

1. **Practice Mindfulness**: Mindfulness techniques, such as meditation and deep breathing exercises, can help manage stress and cravings. Make these habits a regular part of your day-to-day routine.

2. **Educate Yourself**: Read books and attend workshops on mindfulness to enhance your understanding and skills.

3. **Stay Present**: Focus on the present moment and take things one day at a time. This can help reduce anxiety about the future and keep you grounded.

Success stories from individuals who have quit cold turkey highlight the importance of staying active, building a support network, practicing mindfulness, and staying positive. By understanding the pros and cons and learning from others' experiences, you can make an informed decision about whether quitting cold turkey is the right approach for you.

Ultimately, the key to success lies in your determination, preparation, and willingness to seek support when needed. Whether you choose to quit cold turkey or use other methods, the goal is the same: achieving a healthier, smoke-free life.

GRADUAL REDUCTIONS

CREATING A REDUCTION PLAN

Quitting smoking through gradual reduction involves slowly decreasing your nicotine intake over time, rather than stopping all at once. This method can be less intimidating and more manageable for many smokers, providing a structured approach to quitting that can reduce the severity of withdrawal symptoms. To successfully quit through gradual reduction, creating a detailed and personalized reduction plan is essential.

Assess Your Current Smoking Habits

The first step in creating a reduction plan is to assess your current smoking habits. Keep a detailed diary for one week, recording every cigarette you smoke. Note the time of day, your mood, and the circumstances surrounding each cigarette. This information will help you identify patterns and triggers, which are crucial for developing an effective reduction strategy.

Set a Quit Date

Choose a quit date that gives you enough time to gradually reduce your smoking. This date should be realistic and achievable, typically ranging from a few weeks to a few months from when you start the reduction plan. Having a clear end goal in mind provides motivation and a sense of purpose.

Determine Your Reduction Rate

Decide how quickly you want to reduce your smoking. This can be done by cutting down on the number of cigarettes you smoke each day or by delaying the first cigarette of the day. A common approach is to reduce your daily cigarette intake by one or two cigarettes every few days or every week. Alternatively, you might choose to extend the intervals between cigarettes, gradually increasing the time you wait before having your next one.

Create a Schedule

Develop a detailed schedule outlining your reduction plan. This schedule should specify how many cigarettes you will smoke each day and when you will reduce your intake. For example, if you smoke 20 cigarettes a day, your schedule might look like this:

- Week 1: 18 cigarettes per day
- Week 2: 16 cigarettes per day
- Week 3: 14 cigarettes per day
- Week 4: 12 cigarettes per day

And so on, until you reach zero. This schedule provides a clear roadmap and helps you stay on track.

Identify and Replace Triggers

Identify the specific triggers that prompt you to smoke, such as stress, boredom, or social situations. Develop alternative coping strategies to replace smoking when these triggers occur. For example, if you smoke to relieve stress, consider practicing relaxation techniques like deep breathing, meditation, or physical exercise. If boredom is a trigger, find engaging activities or hobbies to keep yourself occupied.

Prepare for Challenges

Anticipate challenges and plan how you will address them. Cravings and withdrawal symptoms are common during the reduction process. Having a plan in place for managing these challenges can help you stay committed to your reduction plan. This might include strategies like drinking water, chewing gum, or practicing mindfulness techniques when cravings strike.

Tracking Your Progress

Tracking your progress is a critical component of a successful gradual reduction plan. Regularly monitoring your smoking habits and celebrating milestones can keep you motivated and provide a sense of accomplishment.

Maintain a Smoking Diary

Continue to keep a smoking diary throughout the reduction process. Record the number of cigarettes you smoke each day, noting any deviations from your reduction schedule. Also, track your cravings and the strategies you use to manage them. This diary will provide valuable insights into your progress and help you identify areas where you might need to adjust your plan.

Use Technology

Consider using technology to assist with tracking your progress. There are numerous mobile apps designed to help people quit smoking. These apps often include features like daily smoking logs, progress charts, and reminders. They can also provide motivational messages and tips for managing cravings.

Set Milestones

Break your overall goal into smaller, achievable milestones. For example, if you start at 20 cigarettes a day, your first milestone might be reducing to 15 cigarettes a day. Celebrate each milestone you reach, whether it's through a small reward or simply acknowledging your achievement. Implementing positive reinforcement can enhance your motivation and self-assurance.

Review and Adjust Your Plan

Regularly review your reduction plan and progress. If you find that a particular reduction rate is too challenging, consider adjusting your schedule to make it more manageable. Flexibility is important; the goal is to continue making progress, even if it's at a slower pace than originally planned.

Seek Support

Share your progress with friends, family, or support groups. Their encouragement and feedback can provide additional motivation and accountability. Consider joining online forums or local support groups where you can connect with others who are also working towards quitting smoking as was said earlier.

Handling Setbacks

Setbacks are a normal part of the quitting process, and handling them effectively is crucial for long-term success. Whether you smoke more cigarettes than planned or experience strong cravings, knowing how to manage setbacks can help you stay on track.

Recognize that Setbacks are Normal

Understand that setbacks are a common part of the quitting journey. Many people who successfully quit smoking have experienced setbacks along the way. Rather than viewing a setback as a failure, see it as an opportunity to learn and adjust your approach.

Identify the Cause

When a setback occurs, take some time to reflect on what triggered it. Was it a stressful event, a social situation, or an emotional response? Identifying the cause can help you develop strategies to prevent similar setbacks in the future.

Adjust Your Plan

If you experience a setback, it might be necessary to adjust your reduction plan. This could involve slowing down your reduction rate, incorporating additional coping strategies, or seeking extra support. The key is to remain flexible and make adjustments that will help you continue progressing towards your goal.

Stay Positive

Always have a positive mindset, even when you encounter setbacks. Remind yourself of the progress you've made and the reasons you want to quit smoking. Positive self-talk and focusing on your achievements can help you stay motivated and resilient.

Seek Professional Help

If you're struggling to handle setbacks on your own, consider seeking professional help. A therapist or counselor who specializes in smoking cessation can provide personalized support and strategies to help you overcome challenges. Support groups and online communities can also offer encouragement and practical advice from others who have faced similar setbacks.

Focus on the Long-Term Goal

Keep your long-term goal in mind: becoming smoke-free. While setbacks can be discouraging, they don't define your entire journey. Focus on the progress you've made and the benefits of quitting smoking. Each day without a cigarette is a step towards a healthier, smoke-free life.

Gradual reduction is a practical and effective approach to quitting smoking for many people. By creating a detailed reduction plan, tracking your progress, and handling setbacks with resilience and flexibility, you can successfully navigate the challenges of quitting. Remember that quitting smoking is a journey, and setbacks are a normal part of that journey. With determination, support, and a positive mindset, you can achieve your goal of becoming smoke-free.

NICOTINE REPLACEMENT THERAPY (NRT)

Nicotine replacement therapy (NRT) serves as an aid to help you kick the smoking habit. It provides small, measured amounts of nicotine to ease the symptoms of withdrawal and cravings. You have a variety of choices and can mix and match these aids. It's wise to consult a healthcare professional before embarking on NRT.

Let's take a closer look:

What's the deal with nicotine replacement therapy (NRT)?

NRT is all about using certain products, such as gum or patches, that deliver small doses of nicotine. This helps to reduce your urge to smoke and the discomfort of withdrawal. Think of it as a supportive medication treatment for those hooked on nicotine from smoking. These NRT options are free from the harmful stuff—like the cancer-causing agents—you get from tobacco smoke.

While NRT tackles the physical tug-of-war of quitting, it doesn't cover the whole quitting landscape, like the mental and social challenges. Quitting smoking is tough, even with NRT's help. But pairing NRT with other approaches, like counseling or a quit-smoking program, can really boost your odds of breaking free for good.

Who should consider NRT?

NRT is tailored for individuals who are strongly hooked on nicotine and determined to quit smoking. Its effectiveness for quitting other forms of tobacco hasn't been as thoroughly researched.

Nicotine, a stimulant found in tobacco, can lead to addiction when your body grows accustomed to a certain nicotine level. This dependency can manifest both physically and psychologically.

You might have a serious nicotine addiction if you:

- Smoke over a pack a day.
- Light up soon after waking.
- Smoke even when you're under the weather.
- Get up to smoke during the night.
- Smoke to fend off withdrawal symptoms.

NRT is generally considered safe for most adults aiming to quit. However, it's not recommended for pregnant individuals or teenagers. Also, if you have liver or kidney problems, NRT might not be safe. Always check with a healthcare provider to see if NRT is a good fit for you.

How does nicotine replacement therapy function?

NRT works by giving you controlled, low doses of nicotine to help manage cravings and withdrawal after you've stopped smoking. NRT products deliver nicotine more slowly and in smaller amounts than cigarettes.

These products include nicotine:

- Gum.
- Lozenges.

- Patches for the skin.
- Inhalers.
- Nasal sprays.

Approved by the FDA for smoking cessation, these products can be harmful if overused or if used while still smoking, as they could lead to nicotine poisoning.

Before diving into NRT, have a chat with a healthcare provider to figure out the most effective strategy for you. Here are some pointers:

- It's suggested to begin NRT either a week or two before you quit or right after you stop smoking.
- Joining a quit-smoking counseling program while on NRT can significantly improve your quitting success.
- The more you smoked, the stronger the initial dose of nicotine you might need.
- Gradually reduce your nicotine dose throughout the NRT process.
- Always store NRT products out of reach of children and pets to prevent accidental poisoning.

Using Nicotine Gum

Nicotine gum is readily available without a prescription. To use it, simply chew the gum until you notice a peppery taste or a tingling sensation, then park it between your cheek and gums for about half an hour. Always stick to the guidelines provided on the packaging, and remember these pointers:

- Hold off on coffee, tea, or acidic drinks like orange juice for 15 minutes before chewing nicotine gum.
- For the initial six weeks of quitting, you might chew a piece every one to two hours to fend off cravings.
- After six weeks, you can cut down to one piece every two to four hours, and eventually to one every four to eight hours.
- Only chew one piece at a time, and aim to quit using the gum within 12 weeks. If you're thinking about using it longer, chat with your healthcare provider first.

Using Nicotine Lozenges

Nicotine lozenges are like hard candy and are available over the counter. Place one in your mouth and let it dissolve slowly, releasing nicotine. You'll likely feel a warm, tingly sensation. Here's how to use them responsibly:

- Generally, you can have one lozenge every one to two hours during the first six weeks after you quit smoking.
- Then, reduce the frequency to one lozenge every two to four hours, and later to one every four to eight hours.
- Remember to stick to just one lozenge at a time.

Using Nicotine Patches

Nicotine patches are another over-the-counter option that you apply to your skin each morning. They deliver a steady nicotine dose throughout the day. Here's the lowdown on patches:

- Patches come in various strengths, so choose the right one based on your smoking habits.
- Typically, you wear a patch for 16 or 24 hours and it's okay to keep it on while showering or bathing.
- Apply the patch to a clean, dry, and hairless area of your upper body, and rotate the application site daily.

Using Nicotine Inhalers

Nicotine inhalers need a prescription. They're not like e-cigarettes; they're FDA-approved for quitting smoking. To use an inhaler:

- Cartridge use and daily limits depend on the brand.
- Take short, shallow puffs – deep inhalation isn't necessary.
- Avoid eating or drinking 15 minutes before and during use.

Using Nicotine Nasal Sprays

Nicotine nasal sprays also require a prescription. They deliver nicotine quickly when sprayed into the nostrils. Here's what to keep in mind:

- Typically, you'll use at least eight doses a day for the first six weeks, not exceeding 40 doses a day.
- Use is most times limited to three months.
- Follow your provider's instructions closely due to the potential for addiction, and discuss any concerns about overuse with them.

Mixing Different NRT Options

Different NRT (Nicotine Replacement Therapy) products work in unique ways, and you might find it beneficial to use a combination to support your effort to quit smoking. A longer-lasting option like a nicotine patch can help reduce withdrawal symptoms, while a quicker-acting solution can address sudden cravings when they arise.

You can pair a long-acting NRT, such as a patch, with a short-acting one like this:

- Nicotine gum with a patch.
- Nicotine lozenges with a patch.
- Nicotine inhaler with a patch.
- Nicotine nasal spray with a patch.

Always consult with your healthcare provider to figure out the safest and most effective way to use multiple NRT products.

Pros and Cons of NRT

What's good about nicotine replacement therapy?

NRT can significantly curb your need to smoke by supplying nicotine in a less harmful form. Research indicates that NRT can boost your odds of kicking the habit by 50% to 70%.

What about the downsides of NRT?

Each NRT option comes with its own set of possible side effects. Make sure to read the instructions and talk to a healthcare professional before starting, so you know what might come up.

Generally, because they contain nicotine, NRT products might lead to:

- Nausea.
- Headaches.
- A quickened heartbeat.

Specifically, nicotine patches can cause:

- Skin irritation.
- Sleep disturbances or vivid dreams.

Nicotine gum might lead to:

- Throat discomfort.
- Mouth ulcers.
- Hiccups.

Nicotine lozenges could cause:

- Hiccups.
- A sore throat.
- Coughing.
- Heartburn.

Nicotine nasal spray side effects (typically short-term) include:

- Irritation in the nose or throat.
- Runny nose.
- Teary eyes.
- Sneezing.
- Coughing.

Nicotine inhalers might cause:

- Coughing.
- Irritation in the mouth or throat.
- Runny nose.
- Upset stomach.

Watch Out for Nicotine Poisoning

It's crucial to use NRT as directed. Overuse or using them while still smoking can lead to nicotine overdose, which is dangerous for kids and pets too.

Early signs of nicotine poisoning include:

- Nausea and vomiting.
- Excessive saliva.
- Stomach pain.
- Sweating.
- A fast heartbeat.
- Quick, deep breathing.
- Lack of coordination, trouble walking, or tremors.
- Headaches.
- Dizziness.
- Seizures.

If you or someone you know has these symptoms, get to an emergency room.

WHAT'S NEXT AFTER NRT?

How long does NRT treatment last?

NRT is usually a short-term aid, with many healthcare providers suggesting a duration of eight to 12 weeks. If you're still struggling with cravings or withdrawal after this period, it's time to discuss other options with your healthcare provider.

What if NRT isn't cutting it for me?

Quitting smoking is often a journey with multiple attempts. If NRT isn't doing the trick, you're not alone. Have a chat with your healthcare provider. They might propose another NRT tactic, varying products, or dosages.

The FDA has greenlit two other non-nicotine prescription meds (varenicline and bupropion) for quitting smoking. Your provider might suggest pairing one of these with NRT.

Tackling the mental and emotional aspects of smoking is also key to quitting for good. Inquire about cessation programs that address these factors. Keep on trying – that's the most important step.

When to Reach Out to Your Doctor

When should I talk to my doctor about NRT?

Before you start NRT, it's wise to get advice from your healthcare provider on the best strategy. If side effects are bothering you or if you're encountering challenges in your quit-smoking journey, reach out to them for support and alternative solutions.

Quitting smoking can lead to feelings of depression or anxiety, whether or not you're using NRT. If these mood changes are persistent or distressing, don't hesitate to speak with your provider or seek help from a mental health professional.

BEHAVIORAL THERAPIES

Behavioral therapies are a cornerstone in the treatment of smoking addiction, helping individuals modify their habits and manage cravings.

These therapies address the psychological aspects of addiction and provide tools to cope with the triggers and stressors that lead to smoking. Among the most effective behavioral therapies for quitting smoking are Cognitive-Behavioral Therapy (CBT), hypnotherapy, and mindfulness and meditation techniques.

COGNITIVE-BEHAVIORAL THERAPY (CBT)

Understanding CBT

CBT is a psychotherapy that aims to change negative thoughts and behaviors through structure and goals. It is based on the concept that our thoughts, feelings, and behaviors are interconnected, and that changing negative thoughts and behaviors can improve emotional regulation and develop coping strategies for dealing with problematic issues, such as smoking addiction.

HOW CBT HELPS IN SMOKING CESSATION

CBT is particularly effective for smoking cessation because it helps individuals understand the triggers and underlying reasons for their smoking behavior. It teaches practical skills to manage cravings, cope with stress, and replace smoking with healthier habits.

1. **Identifying Triggers**: The first step in CBT for smoking cessation is to identify the specific situations, emotions, and thoughts that trigger the urge to smoke. It could involve stress, social settings, or specific times. Recognizing these triggers enables individuals to devise strategies for avoidance or coping.

2. **Challenging Negative Thoughts**: CBT helps individuals challenge and change negative thought patterns that lead to smoking. For example, a smoker might believe that smoking helps them relax. Through CBT, they can learn to recognize this belief as a cognitive distortion and replace it with more accurate thoughts, such as recognizing that smoking actually increases stress in the long term.

3. **Developing Coping Strategies**: CBT teaches practical coping strategies to deal with cravings and stress without smoking. This might include deep breathing exercises, physical activity, or engaging in

hobbies. Learning and practicing these strategies can help reduce the reliance on smoking as a coping mechanism.

4. **Relapse Prevention**: CBT includes techniques for preventing relapse, such as developing a plan for dealing with high-risk situations and building a strong support network. Individuals learn to anticipate challenges and have strategies in place to maintain their smoke-free status.

STRUCTURE OF CBT SESSIONS

CBT for smoking cessation typically involves a series of structured sessions with a trained therapist. These sessions might be conducted individually or in a group setting. Each session has specific goals, such as identifying triggers, practicing coping strategies, and monitoring progress. Homework assignments, such as keeping a smoking diary or practicing relaxation techniques, are often used to reinforce what is learned in sessions.

HYPNOTHERAPY

Understanding Hypnotherapy

Hypnotherapy involves the use of hypnosis to create a state of focused attention and increased susceptibility as a therapeutic technique. The therapist uses hypnosis to guide a person into a relaxed state, making them more open to suggestions. These suggestions can help change their thoughts, feelings, and behaviors related to smoking.

HOW HYPNOTHERAPY HELPS IN SMOKING CESSATION

Hypnotherapy can be effective in smoking cessation by targeting the subconscious mind to alter the perception and habits associated with smoking. The therapist uses suggestions and imagery to help the individual develop a negative association with smoking and a positive association with being smoke-free.

1. **Creating Aversion**: One common approach in hypnotherapy for smoking cessation is to create an aversion to smoking. The therapist

might suggest that cigarettes taste and smell unpleasant, or that smoking makes the individual feel sick. This aversion can reduce the desire to smoke.

2. **Enhancing Motivation**: Hypnotherapy can also enhance motivation to quit by reinforcing the benefits of being smoke-free. The therapist might suggest that the individual feels healthier, happier, and more in control without smoking. These positive suggestions can boost confidence and commitment to quitting.

3. **Addressing Underlying Issues**: Hypnotherapy can help address underlying emotional issues that contribute to smoking, such as anxiety, stress, or low self-esteem. By resolving these issues, individuals may find it easier to quit smoking.

4. **Reducing Withdrawal Symptoms**: Hypnotherapy can be used to reduce the discomfort of withdrawal symptoms. Suggestions might include feeling calm and relaxed, having minimal cravings, and easily handling any discomfort that arises.

STRUCTURE OF HYPNOTHERAPY SESSIONS

Hypnotherapy sessions for smoking cessation typically begin with an initial consultation to discuss the individual's smoking history, goals, and any concerns. The hypnotherapist then guides the individual into a state of relaxation and makes positive suggestions related to quitting smoking. Multiple sessions may be needed to reinforce these suggestions and address any challenges that arise.

MINDFULNESS AND MEDITATION TECHNIQUES

Understanding Mindfulness and Meditation

Mindfulness involves paying attention to the present moment without judgment, while meditation is a practice that trains the mind to achieve a state of calm and focused awareness. Both techniques can be powerful tools in managing stress, cravings, and the emotional aspects of smoking addiction.

How Mindfulness and Meditation Help in Smoking Cessation

Mindfulness and meditation help individuals develop greater awareness of their thoughts, emotions, and bodily sensations. This heightened awareness can break the automatic patterns of smoking and provide alternative ways to cope with cravings and stress.

1. **Mindful Awareness of Cravings**: Mindfulness teaches individuals to observe their cravings without immediately reacting to them. By noticing the sensations and thoughts associated with cravings, individuals can learn to sit with the discomfort and let it pass rather than giving in to the urge to smoke.

2. **Stress Reduction**: Meditation techniques, such as deep breathing and progressive muscle relaxation, can reduce stress and anxiety, which are common triggers for smoking. By cultivating a state of calm and relaxation, individuals are less likely to reach for a cigarette as a way to cope.

3. **Breaking Automatic Patterns**: Mindfulness helps individuals become aware of the automatic patterns that lead to smoking. For example, they might notice that they light a cigarette without thinking whenever they finish a meal. By bringing awareness to these patterns, they can consciously choose a different response.

4. **Promoting Self-Compassion**: Mindfulness and meditation foster a sense of self-compassion, which can be particularly helpful in dealing with the challenges of quitting. Rather than criticizing themselves for cravings or setbacks, individuals learn to treat themselves with kindness and understanding, which supports long-term success.

Practicing Mindfulness and Meditation

There are various ways to incorporate mindfulness and meditation into a smoking cessation plan:

- **Mindful Breathing**: Focus on your breath, observing the sensation of the air entering and leaving your body. Use this technique whenever you experience cravings or stress.
- **Body Scan Meditation**: Progressively focus on different parts of your body, noticing any tension or discomfort. This practice can

help you become more aware of the physical sensations associated with cravings.

- **Mindfulness-Based Stress Reduction (MBSR):** Consider enrolling in an MBSR program, which combines mindfulness meditation and yoga to reduce stress and improve overall well-being.
- **Guided Meditations**: Use guided meditation recordings specifically designed for smoking cessation. These recordings can provide structure and support as you develop your meditation practice.

Behavioral therapies such as Cognitive-Behavioral Therapy (CBT), hypnotherapy, and mindfulness and meditation techniques offer effective strategies for quitting smoking by addressing the psychological aspects of addiction. CBT helps individuals identify triggers, challenge negative thoughts, and develop coping strategies. Hypnotherapy targets the subconscious mind to alter perceptions and habits related to smoking. Mindfulness and meditation promote awareness, stress reduction, and self-compassion, providing tools to manage cravings and emotional challenges.

Each of these therapies can be used individually or in combination, depending on your preferences and needs. By incorporating behavioral therapies into your smoking cessation plan, you can develop the skills and resilience needed to achieve and maintain a smoke-free life.

Alternative Approaches

HERBAL REMEDIES AND NATURAL SUPPLEMENTS

Herbal remedies and natural supplements have been used for centuries in various cultures to aid in health and wellness, including smoking cessation. While scientific evidence supporting their efficacy may vary, many people find these alternative approaches beneficial either as primary strategies or complementary to other cessation methods. Understanding the potential benefits and how to use these remedies can provide additional tools in the journey to quit smoking.

Herbal Remedies

1. **Lobelia (Lobelia inflata)**

Lobelia, also known as Indian tobacco, is one of the most commonly used herbs for quitting smoking. It contains lobeline, a substance believed to mimic the effects of nicotine on the brain. Remember this: "It helps relieve withdrawal symptoms and cravings".

> ➢ **How to Use**: Lobelia is available in various forms, including tinctures, capsules, and teas. It's crucial to follow dosage recommendations, as high doses can be toxic. Before using, it's best to consult a healthcare provider.

2. **St. John's Wort (Hypericum perforatum)**

St. John's Wort is traditionally used to treat depression and anxiety, which can be beneficial during the stressful period of quitting smoking. Its mood-stabilizing effects may help manage the emotional ups and downs associated with nicotine withdrawal.

> ➢ **How to Use**: St. John's Wort is commonly available in capsules, tablets, and teas. As it can interact with other medications, it's

essential to consult with a healthcare provider before starting this supplement.

3. Valerian (Valeriana officinalis)

Valerian root is often used for its calming and sedative properties. It can help manage the anxiety and insomnia that sometimes accompany smoking cessation.

- ➤ **How to Use**: Valerian can be taken as a tea, tincture, or in capsule form. It is typically used before bedtime to aid sleep and reduce anxiety.

4. Ginseng (Panax ginseng)

Ginseng is known for its energy-boosting properties and its ability to help the body handle stress. It can support the body during the withdrawal phase and reduce cravings by stabilizing blood sugar levels.

- ➤ **How to Use:** Ginseng is available in powders, capsules, and teas. Daily supplementation can help mitigate the energy lows and stress associated with quitting smoking.

Natural Supplements

1. **Vitamin C**

Vitamin C can help repair the damage caused by smoking. It also helps to flush nicotine out of the body faster, reducing cravings more quickly.

> ➤ **How to Use**: Increase your intake of Vitamin C-rich foods like oranges, strawberries, and bell peppers, or take a Vitamin C supplement as directed.

2. **B Vitamins**

B Vitamins, particularly B6 and B12, support the nervous system and can help manage the stress and mood swings that often come with quitting smoking.

> ➤ **How to Use**: Take a B-complex supplement or increase your intake of foods rich in B vitamins, such as whole grains, eggs, and leafy greens.

3. Magnesium

Magnesium helps regulate neurotransmitters in the brain, promoting relaxation and aiding in sleep. It can help reduce the anxiety and irritability associated with nicotine withdrawal.

> - **How to Use**: Magnesium supplements are available in various forms, including tablets and powders. Foods high in magnesium, such as nuts, seeds, and leafy greens, can also be included in your diet.

Combining Herbal Remedies and Supplements

Using a combination of herbal remedies and natural supplements can provide a more comprehensive approach to smoking cessation. For example, combining the stress-relief benefits of St. John's Wort with the calming effects of valerian can help manage both the emotional and physical aspects of nicotine withdrawal. Don't forget to consult with a healthcare provider before combining supplements to prevent any potential interactions.

THE ROLE OF EXERCISE AND NUTRITION

Exercise and nutrition play a crucial role in the process of quitting smoking. Regular physical activity and a balanced diet can help manage withdrawal symptoms, reduce cravings, and improve overall health. Incorporating these elements into your smoking cessation plan can enhance your chances of success.

Exercise

1. **Benefits of Exercise for Smoking Cessation**

- **Reduces Cravings**: Exercise stimulates the release of endorphins, which can reduce nicotine cravings and improve mood.
- **Manages Stress**: Physical activity is an effective way to reduce stress and anxiety, common triggers for smoking.
- **Improves Lung Function**: Regular exercise can help improve lung capacity and function, aiding in the detoxification process.

- **Promotes Weight Management**: Exercise helps control weight, addressing concerns about weight gain after quitting smoking.

2. Types of Exercise

- **Aerobic Exercise**: Activities like walking, running, swimming, and cycling are effective for cardiovascular health and lung function.
- **Strength Training**: Building muscle through weightlifting or bodyweight exercises can improve overall fitness and metabolism.
- **Flexibility and Relaxation:** Practices such as yoga and Pilates enhance flexibility, reduce stress, and promote relaxation.

3. Creating an Exercise Routine

- **Start Slow**: Begin with moderate activities and gradually increase intensity and duration.
- **Find Enjoyable Activities**: Choose exercises you enjoy to stay motivated and consistent.
- **Set Realistic Goals**: Establish achievable goals to track progress and maintain motivation.

- Avoid boredom and improve overall fitness by combining various types of exercise.

Nutrition

1. The Importance of a Healthy Diet

A balanced diet supports the body's ability to heal and adapt to the changes that come with quitting smoking. Proper nutrition can help manage cravings, improve mood, and enhance overall health.

2. Key Nutrients

- **Antioxidants**: Foods rich in antioxidants, such as fruits and vegetables, help repair the damage caused by smoking.
- **Protein**: Adequate protein intake supports muscle repair and growth, especially important if you are incorporating exercise.
- **Complex Carbohydrates**: Whole grains, legumes, and starchy vegetables provide sustained energy and help stabilize blood sugar levels.

- **Healthy Fats**: Include sources of omega-3 fatty acids, such as fish, flaxseeds, and walnuts, to support brain health and reduce inflammation.
- **Hydration**: Staying hydrated helps flush toxins from the body and can reduce cravings

PART IV: STAYING SMOKE-FREE

MANAGING CRAVINGS AND WITHDRAWAL SYMPTOMS

It is not only a matter of stopping smoking when one desires to quit. This involves managing the cravings and withdrawal symptoms that occur as part of freeing oneself from nicotine addiction. Therefore, understanding cravings, developing effective coping strategies, and planning for long-term withdrawal management are some of the important elements in quitting successfully.

Understanding Cravings

1. The Nature of Nicotine Addiction

Nicotine is the addictive substance in cigarettes that creates a dependency both physically and psychologically. Whenever you smoke, nicotine passes swiftly into your blood stream and travels to your brain where it causes the release of dopamine-a transmitter associated with pleasurable feelings. As time goes by, episodes of this chemical increase get ingrained in your brain leading to an addiction cycle.

Key Points:

- Nicotine dependence involves physical and psychological addiction.
- Cravings are triggered by the absence of nicotine in the body.
- Knowledge about cravings can be demystified through understanding addiction biology.

2. Triggers for Cravings

Cravings are usually brought on by certain situations, emotions or habits. These stimuli differ from person to person but include;

Key Points:

3. **Situational Triggers**: Activities/environments related to smoking (e.g., having coffee, taking breaks at work).
4. **Emotional Triggers**: Feelings like stress, anxiety or boredom can prompt one to feel the urge to smoke.
5. **Social Triggers**: Among smokers or in settings where smoking occurs frequently.

Some of these has been talked about earlier or later in this book.

3. Cravings in Terms of Duration and Intensity

Normally, cravings will hit their peak within the first few days of quitting and dwindle gradually over time. However, sometimes they may still come up after months or even years have gone by since you last smoked, especially in places that were strongly connected with smoking.

Key Points:

- For most people, cravings do not last longer than a couple of minutes.
- Over time cravings become less intense.
- Expecting unexpected pangs can help you deal with them better.

EFFECTIVE COPING STRATEGIES

1. Behavioral Techniques
2. Cognitive Strategies
3. Pharmacological Aids
4. Support Systems

LONG-TERM WITHDRAWAL MANAGEMENT

Maintaining motivation

Long-term success in quitting smoking depends heavily on staying motivated.

Key Points:

• **Milestones**: Recognize and celebrate your progress (be it a week, month or year) without cigarette.

• **Keep track of gains**: Maintain a diary log of the positive changes you note in terms of your health, financial position and general well-being.

• **Gain more knowledge**: Make sure that you are always knowledgeable about the benefits of quitting smoking and perils of continuing to smoke.

Avoiding Relapse

It is important to stay watchful and equipped to face possible challenges if one wants to prevent relapse from occurring.

Key Points:

- **High-Risk Situations**: Be aware when and where you may be tempted to smoke and plan how to handle them.
- **Create New Habits**: Establish new ways of doing things that do not involve smoking.
- **Stress Management**: Look for healthy methods through which stress can be handled including exercise, meditation or hobbies among others.

Long-Term Health Strategies

Adopting an overall healthy lifestyle can aid in maintaining one's smoke-free status thereby improving their general well-being too.

Key Points:

- **Regular Exercise**: Make physical activities part of your daily program so as to reduce stress levels while also promoting good health at all times.
- **Healthy Eating Habits**: Balanced diet should be consumed in order for the recovery process from effects brought by cigarettes takes place properly;

- **Sleep and Rest**: Ensure you get enough sleep and rest so that your body can heal and handle stress well.

Continued Support

Even after you have quit smoking, ongoing support can help you remain dedicated to living a smoke free life.

Key Points:

- **Periodic Check-Ins**: Schedule regular check-ins with your healthcare provider to monitor your progress and address any concerns.
- **Stay Connected**: Maintain connections with your support group or find new ones to keep yourself accountable.
- **Reinforce Your Commitment:** Remind yourself regularly of the reasons you quit and the benefits you've gained.

Managing cravings and withdrawal symptoms is an important part of quitting smoking. By understanding what cravings are all about, employing effective coping mechanisms, and planning for long-term withdrawal management, quitting becomes easier. Stay committed, seek support, every step counts towards a healthier future without cigarettes.

STAYING SMOKE-FREE

Kicking the smoking habit is a tremendous accomplishment, yet the real challenge often lies in sticking to a non-smoking lifestyle. To keep from falling back into old habits, it's vital to stay alert for any signs of a potential slip-up, remain steadfast in your commitment, and navigate through tempting scenarios with skill. These steps are key to continuing your smoke-free journey.

SPOTTING EARLY RED FLAGS

Staying alert for early signs of a possible smoking relapse is crucial to keeping up your smoke-free life. Catching these hints early on means you can act fast to stop a minor wobble from turning into a major setback. Paying attention to what sets off your cravings can help you stay on course.

MENTAL AND EMOTIONAL CLUES

1. **Surging Stress and Anxiety**

Feeling more stressed or anxious than usual can push you toward lighting up again. If life's pressures start piling up, whether from work or personal issues, watch out—it could be a sign you're veering toward old habits.

How to Manage: Work stress-busting activities into your day, like deep breathing, meditation, yoga, or exercise.

2. Moodiness and Quick Temper

If you're riding an emotional rollercoaster or getting ticked off more easily, it might be a sign you're missing nicotine's calming effect. These mood changes can weaken your resolve to stay smoke-free.

How to Manage: Keep your lifestyle balanced with enough sleep, regular physical activity, and a healthy diet. If emotions run high, consider chatting with a therapist or counselor.

3. Feeling Swamped

When life's demands feel like too much, you might think about smoking to cope. Catching yourself feeling swamped is a signal to take action against a potential smoking relapse.

How to Manage: Tackle tasks in small steps, sort out your priorities, and don't shy away from asking for help.

BEHAVIORAL RED FLAGS

1. Cravings and Urges

Noticing a spike in your desire to smoke is a glaring red flag. Cravings can pop up due to stress, social settings, or even at particular times of the day.

How to Manage: Keep a log of when cravings hit to find patterns. Have a go-to list of distractions for when the urge to smoke strikes.

2. Making Excuses for Smoking

If you catch yourself making excuses to smoke, like "just one won't hurt" or "I can quit again later," it's a warning that you might be slipping.

How to Manage: Remind yourself why you quit and the perks of living smoke-free. Pump yourself up with positive self-talk to combat these excuses.

3. Shying Away from Support

If you're skipping out on friends or meetings that help you stay off cigarettes, it's a sign you might be heading for a relapse.

How to Manage: Keep in touch with your support circle. Regularly attend support group sessions or counseling to keep your commitment strong.

ENVIRONMENTAL HAZARDS

1. Hanging in Smoking Zones

Spending more time in places where smoking is common can tempt you to join in.

How to Manage: Stay away from these spots when you can. Seek out new, smoke-free surroundings that support your quit mission.

2. Time with Smokers

Being around friends who smoke, especially if you used to join them, can be a big trigger.

How to Manage: Share your goal to stay smoke-free and ask for their backing. If needed, limit time in smoky places.

3. Seeing Smoking Gear

Coming across cigarettes, lighters, or ashtrays can stir up cravings.

How to Manage: Clear out any smoking gear from your space. Replace them with things that encourage a healthy lifestyle.

STICKING TO YOUR GUTS

Staying true to your smoke-free path means consistently applying strategies that support your decision. These tactics help you stay on track, fend off temptations, and keep your health front and center.

Goal-Setting

1. Short-Term Targets

Having bite-sized goals can keep you driven and give you little victories to celebrate along the way.

Examples: Aim to be smoke-free for a week, then a month, and so on. Reward yourself after each milestone with something you love.

2. Long-Term Ambitions

Thinking about the big picture and the lasting advantages of quitting smoking can help you stay motivated.

Examples: Imagine the health improvements, money saved, and new activities you'll enjoy without smoking's hold on you.

Routine Building

1. Daily Structure

A well-planned day can keep you too busy to think about smoking and cut down on downtime, which might trigger cravings.

Tips: Fill your schedule with activities that boost your health and happiness, like working out, diving into hobbies, and hanging out with supportive folks.

2. Healthy Habits

Swapping smoking for wholesome habits can boost your health and lessen the urge to light up.

Examples: Drink lots of water, eat nutritious meals, get active, and try relaxation techniques.

Positive Encouragement

1. Rewarding Yourself

Treating yourself for staying smoke-free can motivate you and give you milestones to look forward to.

Examples: Indulge in a movie, a new book, or a nice meal when you hit your goals. Save the cash you'd have spent on cigarettes for bigger treats, like a holiday.

2. Cheering Yourself On

Keeping your spirits up with positive self-talk can help you stay firm in your decision to quit.

Tips: Boost your morale with affirmations like "I'm strong enough to stay smoke-free," "I choose health over smoking," and "I'm proud of how far I've come."

Supportive Actions

1. Joining Support Circles

Finding a community in support groups can offer companionship and accountability. Sharing your journey with those who get it can be a huge help.

Perks: Get cheered on, learn new coping methods, and pick up tips from those who've successfully quit.

2. Professional Guidance

Getting help from a counselor or therapist can give you specialized support and strategies that fit your situation. They can help you tackle deeper reasons you might smoke.

Perks: Benefit from expert advice, tailored tactics, and emotional backing.

MANAGING TEMPTING TIMES

Dealing with tricky situations is key to avoiding a smoking relapse. These moments can bring on strong cravings, so having a game plan is essential.

Social Scenes

1. Festivities and Hangouts

Socializing where alcohol flows or cigarettes are in sight can make saying no to smoking tough.

Game Plan: Think ahead by bringing along non-alcoholic drinks and healthy bites. Let your friends know you're committed to not smoking and ask for their help.

2. Work Functions

Office events can be risky, especially if coworkers smoke or there's stress in the air. These settings can make you want to smoke to unwind.

Game Plan: Take breaks to refresh yourself and practice calming breaths. Stick with nonsmoking colleagues for support during these times.

Emotional Challenges

1. Stress Management

Stress can be a major smoking trigger. Learning to handle it well can keep you from reaching for a cigarette when times get tough.

Game Plan: Turn to stress-relief techniques like meditation, yoga, exercise, or hobbies that calm and captivate you.

2. Navigating Negative Feelings

Dealing with anger, sadness, or frustration can make you crave the comfort of a smoke.

Game Plan: Get to the heart of what's bugging you by talking to a trusted pal or seeking counseling. Find activities that boost your mood and offer solace.

Routine Disruptions

1. **Traveling**

Travel can throw off your habits and introduce new triggers. Being out of your comfort zone can make smoking seem tempting.

Game Plan: Plan trips with health in mind and choose smoke-free spots. Bring along wholesome snacks and drink water to keep cravings at bay.

2. **Big Life Shifts**

Major changes like moving, starting a new job, or going through a significant personal event can be stressful and spark a smoking urge.

Game Plan: Get ready for these shifts by building a solid support network and focusing on self-care. Concentrate on the positives of the change and your smoke-free commitment.

CULTIVATING A HEALTH-CONSCIOUS LIFESTYLE

ADOPTING NEW PATTERNS

Giving up smoking is a significant leap toward a healthier existence. To preserve this improvement, it's essential to cultivate new, beneficial routines that take the place of the detrimental ones. These new practices do more than just occupy the space left by smoking; they enhance overall health and diminish the chance of returning to old habits.

Grasping the Mechanics of Habit Development

1. **The Mechanics Behind Habits**

Habits are behaviors that become automatic through repetition. Grasping the mechanics behind habit formation aids in establishing new ones to take the place of smoking, involving a cue, a behavior, and a reward.

- **Cue**: An event that triggers the action.
- **Routine**: The action itself.
- **Reward**: The positive feedback that comes after the action.

2. Dismantling Old Habits

To break the smoking habit, one must pinpoint the cues that spark the urge to smoke and seek out healthier behaviors to act as replacements.

Example: If stress prompts smoking, adopt a stress-relief method like deep breathing or a quick stroll instead.

Creating Wholesome Routines

1. Morning Rituals

A positive morning ritual can set an upbeat mood for the day and lessen the temptation to smoke. Include activities that foster well-being and keep cravings at bay.

Examples: Engage in morning exercise, enjoy a nutritious breakfast, meditate, or take a brisk walk to start your day invigorated and stress-free.

2. Breaks Throughout the Day

Those who have quit smoking often miss the routine of taking smoking breaks. Swapping these out with wholesome activities can maintain a sense of structure and offer similar benefits, minus the health hazards.

Examples: opt for a brief walk, practice mindfulness, do some stretching, or savor a piece of fruit as healthier alternatives.

3. Evening Customs

Concluding the day with calming activities can help alleviate stress and curb nighttime cravings.

Examples: Unwind by reading, practicing yoga, journaling, or spending time with family and friends.

Partaking in New Pastimes

1. Physical Activities

Incorporating physical activities into your daily life not only boosts health but also distracts from the urge to smoke.

Examples: Get involved in team sports, hiking, biking, swimming, or gardening for both enjoyment and health benefits. Most of these were said before and repeated to understand better on how to make good use and when it is mostly effective.

2. Creative Endeavors

Creative pursuits can offer a sense of accomplishment and occupy time that might have been spent smoking.

Examples: Try your hand at painting, writing, making music, or crafting for pleasure and personal fulfillment.

3. Social Engagements

Having a support network is vital for sticking to a smoke-free life. Engaging in social activities can bolster relationships and provide a supportive community.

Examples: Get involved in clubs, attend community gatherings, or join group activities like book clubs or cooking classes to foster a sense of community and belonging.

Upholding Regularity

1. Setting Attainable Goals

Pursuing realistic and achievable goals can help maintain regularity. Smaller, manageable objectives are more enduring and less daunting.

Examples: Begin with aims such as exercising three times weekly, eating five daily servings of fruits and vegetables, or dedicating 15 minutes to a hobby each day.

2. Monitoring Advancements

Keeping track of your progress can offer motivation and a feeling of achievement. Using a journal or apps to monitor habits can be helpful.

Examples: Record your daily exercise, eating habits, and any cravings or triggers in a journal. Celebrate milestones and advancements.

3. Refining Habits

Staying adaptable is crucial for sustaining new habits. Modify your routines to keep them engaging and effective.

Examples: If a particular workout becomes tedious, try something new. If your morning routine needs refreshing, add new elements like varied breakfast choices or different exercises.

THE SIGNIFICANCE OF NUTRITION AND PHYSICAL ACTIVITY

A nutritious diet and consistent physical activity are essential for a healthful lifestyle, especially when giving up smoking. These elements not only enhance physical health but also aid mental well-being, making it easier to resist the urge to smoke.

Advantages of a Nutritious Diet

1. **Nutritional Reinforcement**

A well-balanced diet delivers vital nutrients that help the body recover from the damage inflicted by smoking. Foods rich in nutrients aid in tissue repair, bolster immune function, and elevate energy levels.

Key Nutrients: Vitamins C and E, beta-carotene, and other antioxidants in fruits and vegetables aid lung tissue repair. Omega-3 fatty acids from fish and flaxseeds support heart health.

2. Managing Body Weight

Weight gain concerns are common when quitting smoking. A balanced diet aids in weight control by providing necessary nutrients without excess calories.

Tips: Practice portion control, steer clear of processed foods, and opt for whole foods like fruits, veggies, lean proteins, and whole grains.

3. Mood and Energy Regulation

Certain foods can affect mood and energy, helping to manage withdrawal symptoms and diminish cravings.

Tips: Include complex carbohydrates like whole grains for sustained energy. Foods high in tryptophan, such as turkey and bananas, can elevate mood.

Incorporating Consistent Exercise

1. Physical Health Gains

Exercise enhances cardiovascular health, lung capacity, and overall fitness, counterbalancing the negative effects of smoking.

Activities: Aerobic exercises like walking, jogging, cycling, and swimming are especially good for heart and lung health.

2. Mental Health Perks

Regular exercise reduces stress, anxiety, and depression, which are frequent smoking triggers. Physical activity releases endorphins, boosting mood and providing a natural euphoria.

Activities: Yoga, Pilates, and mindfulness practices like tai chi can lower stress and sharpen mental focus.

3. Weight Control

Physical activity helps burn calories and build muscle, contributing to weight management and reducing the risk of weight gain post-smoking cessation.

Activities: Engage in strength training, interval workouts, and sports to build muscle and maintain a healthy weight.

Cultivating a Balanced Way of Life

1. Merging Diet and Exercise

A comprehensive approach that merges diet and exercise is most effective for creating a health-conscious lifestyle. These components complement one another and boost overall health.

Tips: Coordinate meals with your workout schedule to ensure proper energy and recuperation. Stay hydrated and consider meal timing in relation to physical activity.

2. Implementing Gradual Modifications

Incremental changes are more enduring than abrupt ones. Gradually introducing healthy foods and exercise into your routine can ease the transition.

Tips: Start by adding more veggies to your dishes or including brief walks in your day. Slowly increase the intensity and duration of your workouts and make healthier food choices over time.

3. **Maintaining Motivation**

Keeping motivated is key to upholding a balanced lifestyle. Setting objectives, tracking progress, and celebrating accomplishments can keep you driven.

Tips: Set practical, attainable goals, such as trying a new vegetable each week or boosting your daily steps. Don't forget to reward yourself for your progress with non-food treats.

EMBRACING THE DELIGHTS OF A NON-SMOKING EXISTENCE

Embracing a smoke-free life means finding new sources of joy and engaging in activities that bring happiness and satisfaction. Adopting a healthier lifestyle not only improves physical health but also enriches mental and emotional well-being.

Pursuing New Interests

1. Venturing into Hobbies

Exploring new hobbies and interests can bring joy and a sense of achievement. These activities can occupy the time once spent on smoking and open doors to personal growth.

Examples: Dive into gardening, painting, photography, cooking, or learning to play an instrument for rewarding and pleasurable experiences.

2. Travel and Adventure

Travel and adventure offer fresh experiences and viewpoints. Exploring unfamiliar places and cultures can provide excitement and a feeling of achievement.

Examples: Organize trips to destinations on your Wishlist, engage in new outdoor activities like kayaking, and immerse yourself in different cultures.

3. Volunteering and Community Engagement

Contributing to the community and helping others can offer a sense of purpose and joy. Volunteering allows you to make a meaningful impact and connect with others who share your values.

Examples: Offer your time at local shelters, join in community clean-ups, or become part of organizations that champion causes you're passionate about.

Fostering Relationships

1. Strengthening Family Ties

Quitting smoking can enhance family relationships. Invest quality time with loved ones to build stronger, healthier bonds.

Examples: Organize family activities, participate in shared interests, and communicate openly about your quitting journey and achievements.

2. Developing New Friendships

Joining interest-based groups and clubs can lead to new friendships. A network of non-smoking friends can reinforce your commitment to a smoke-free life.

Examples: Participate in hobby-related groups, attend local happenings, or sign up for classes and workshops to meet new people and establish meaningful relationships.

Adopting a Positive Attitude

1. Cultivating Thankfulness

Cultivating gratitude helps you appreciate the positive aspects of life. Regularly acknowledging what you're thankful for can enhance your general well-being.

Tips: Maintain a gratitude diary, jot down three things you're thankful for each day, and show appreciation to others.

2. Mindfulness and Meditation Practices

Mindfulness and meditation can keep you grounded and appreciative of the present. These practices reduce stress and promote a clear mind.

Tips: Dedicate daily time for meditation, practice mindful breathing, and participate in activities that encourage mindfulness.

3. Embracing Positive Self-Talk

Adopting positive self-talk through affirmations can bolster a mindset that's aligned with a smoke-free lifestyle. Affirming your strengths can enhance self-esteem and promote optimism.

Suggestions: Compile a roster of affirmations like "I am resilient and free from smoking," "I opt for wellness and joy," and "I take pride in my journey." Make it a habit to recite them daily, particularly when times get tough.

Celebration of Success

1. Recognizing Achievements

Take the time to celebrate every achievement, no matter the size. Acknowledging your strides helps maintain motivation and gives you a sense of pride.

Ideas: Commemorate the anniversary of your quitting date, honor the intervals of being smoke-free, and treat yourself for hitting key achievements.

2. Sharing Your Story

By sharing your smoke-free journey, you can offer support and become a source of inspiration. Your story might encourage others to embark on their journey to quit smoking.

Ideas: Start a blog, engage in online communities or support networks, or get involved in local events to spread your message and motivate others.

3. Contemplating Your Journey

Regularly reflect on your journey and the positive shifts in your life since quitting. This reflection can offer perspective and strengthen your dedication to remaining smoke-free.

Suggestions: Keep a diary to track your experiences, ponder the hurdles you've surmounted, and acknowledge the health and happiness gains.

Envisioning a Brighter Future

1. Crafting Long-Term Aims

Crafting long-term objectives gives you a clear path and encourages you to stick to a smoke-free existence. Your goals should mirror your dreams and the life you wish to lead.

Ideas: Your aims might include sustaining a healthy way of life, achieving personal or professional milestones, and continuously enhancing your physical and mental health.

2. Imagining Your Triumph

Using visualization can aid in maintaining focus on your ambitions. Picturing your triumph can solidify constructive habits and fuel your drive.

Suggestions: Assemble a vision board filled with visuals and phrases that resonate with your ambitions. Dedicate moments each day to envisioning your triumphs and the perks of a smoke-free existence.

3. Seeking Inspiration

Seek out inspiration to remain driven and true to your aspirations. Inspiration can be drawn from a myriad of sources like literature, audio content, mentors, or personal idols.

Ideas: Delve into literature or podcasts about personal growth and wellness, connect with mentors who exemplify your ideal lifestyle, and look up to figures who spark your enthusiasm.

PART V: STORIES OF SUCCESS AND INSPIRATION

INSPIRING STORIES OF QUITTING SMOKING

Conversations with Those Who've Quit

Hearing from those who've successfully quit smoking can be incredibly motivating and provide real-world advice on how to navigate the quitting process. These narratives shine a light on the obstacles, tactics, and victories experienced by individuals who have triumphed over their nicotine dependence. Engaging with former smokers through interviews allows us to grasp the varied routes people take to become smoke-free and the profound personal changes that ensue.

Interview 1: Sarah's Escape from Smoking

1. Background and Early Struggles

At 42, Sarah, a marketing professional, began smoking in her teens, initially for social reasons, but soon found herself hooked, smoking a pack daily by her mid-20s. Despite making numerous attempts to quit, experiencing stress and being in social settings often led to a relapse.

Quote: "I lost track of how many times I attempted to quit, but the demands of my job and socializing with friends always pulled me back in."

2. Moment of Change

Sarah's perspective shifted when her father was diagnosed with lung cancer. Seeing him battle the disease made her aware of smoking's dangers and spurred her to quit for her and her family's sake.

"My dad's battle with cancer was a reality check for me. I knew I needed to stop, not just for myself but for my loved ones as well."

3. Quitting Tactics and Support

She looked for guidance from a therapist and became part of a support group. Sarah also used nicotine replacement therapy (NRT) and leaned on a supportive network of friends and family who cheered her on.

Quote: "Joining the support group was pivotal. Sharing my story and listening to others made me feel I wasn't alone."

4. Post-Quitting Life

Post-quitting, Sarah experienced marked health benefits and a better sense of well-being. She took up running, discovered new stress-relief methods like yoga and meditation, and became more active.

Quote: "Quitting smoking is the best decision I've ever made." I'm fitter, more content, and feel I have more control over my life."

Interview 2: Michael's Non-Smoking Journey

1. Background and Hurdles

Michael, a 35-year-old software developer, picked up smoking in college to deal with the academic load. Over time, it became a hard-to-shake habit. His quitting attempts often failed due to work stress and a lack of support.

Quote: "Cigarettes became my stress-buster. Whenever work piled up, I'd find myself smoking."

2. Choosing to Quit

The catalyst for quitting was his wife's pregnancy. Concerned about his family's well-being, he decided to quit to be a healthy example for his child.

Quote: "Becoming a dad changed everything. I wanted to set a healthy example for my kid."

3. Quit Plan and Resources

Michael combined various strategies, including a quit-smoking app, nicotine patches, and therapy. He also started exercising regularly and practicing mindfulness for stress relief.

Quote: "The app was a lifesaver. It kept track of my progress, gave daily advice, and kept me driven. Therapy also taught me how to handle stress without cigarettes."

4. **Benefits of Quitting**

Quitting smoking significantly improved Michael's health and personal connections. He gained energy, suffered fewer breathing problems, and strengthened his relationship with his wife and child.

Quote: "I'm reborn. I have the energy to play with my kid and I'm more engaged in my relationships."

Interview 3: Emma's Breakthrough

1. **Background and Initial Tries**

Emma, a 50-year-old educator, began smoking in her 20s. Despite various attempts to quit, withdrawal symptoms and social situations often led her back to smoking.

Quote: " Kicking the habit was tough. I might go a few weeks smoke-free, but a social event or a stressful situation would always pull me back in.

2. Push to Quit

A severe case of bronchitis was Emma's turning point. Realizing the damage smoking was doing to her health, she committed to quitting permanently.

Quote: "Getting so sick with bronchitis really made me re-think my priorities. I can't keep pushing myself so hard and neglecting my health".

3. Successful Methods and Support

Emma tried acupuncture and hypnotherapy, which to her surprise, were effective. She also joined an online support group and began documenting her journey and feelings.

Quote: "I was skeptical about acupuncture and hypnotherapy initially, but they really cut down my cravings. The online group was also a major source of inspiration."

4. Life Beyond Smoking

Quitting led to significant health and lifestyle improvements for Emma. She became more physically active, lost weight, and felt a surge in vitality.

Quote: "Quitting smoking has given me a new lease on life. I'm healthier, more energetic, and optimistic about my future."

Sarah, Michael, and Emma's stories underscore the various motivations and approaches that can culminate in successful smoking cessation. Their experiences prove that with the right combination of support, resources, and resolve, breaking free from addiction and embracing a smoke-free existence is within reach.

INSIGHTS FROM THEIR EXPERIENCES

Drawing from the experiences of those who've quit smoking can offer vital lessons for others embarking on their own quitting journey. These insights stress the significance of commitment, support networks, and custom-tailored approaches to conquering addiction. By understanding their paths, we can learn what to anticipate, how to persist, and what strategies may be most effective.

Lesson 1: Motivation's Role

1. Discovering Your 'Why'

A compelling personal reason is key to quitting smoking. Whether it's for better health, family, or personal aspirations, a strong motive can fuel your efforts and keep you steadfast.

Example: Sarah was driven by her father's illness, while Michael's motivation stemmed from fatherhood. These profound reasons kept their focus sharp.

2. Goal-Setting

Defining clear, attainable goals can offer direction and motivation. Break your quitting process into smaller targets and celebrate each success.

Tip: Aim for goals like cutting down daily cigarette intake, achieving a week, then a month, and then longer smoke-free stretches.

Lesson 2: Support's Significance

1. Creating a Support Circle

A robust support network is vital for quitting. Support from loved ones, groups, and counselors can offer encouragement, accountability, and useful tips.

Example: Sarah's local group was a major support, while Michael found therapy and his spouse's support invaluable.

2. Professional Assistance

Professional guidance, like therapy or counseling, can provide tailored strategies and coping skills. Therapists can help tackle underlying issues tied to smoking habits.

Tip: Don't hesitate to seek professional help from those specializing in smoking cessation.

Lesson 3: Tailored Strategies

1. Custom Approaches

There is no one-size-fits-all solution, as effectiveness can vary from person to person. Whether it's NRT, hypnotherapy, acupuncture, or mindfulness, finding the right fit for you is crucial.

Example: Emma was successful with acupuncture and hypnotherapy, while Michael found a quit-smoking app and mindfulness helpful.

2. Combining Methods

Using a mix of techniques can boost your chances of quitting. A blend of behavioral therapy, support groups, and lifestyle changes can offer comprehensive assistance.

Tip: Try different strategy combinations to discover what suits you best.

Lesson 4: Handling Triggers and Urges

1. Recognizing Triggers

Knowing your triggers is essential for managing cravings. Stress, social settings, or certain times can be cues. Identifying these helps you devise strategies to handle or avoid them.

Tip: Use a journal to record your triggers and strategize on managing or evading them.

2. Healthy Alternatives

Finding healthier alternatives can aid in craving management. Engaging in physical activities, hobbies, and relaxation techniques can replace smoking.

Example: Sarah took to running and yoga, which helped her tackle stress and maintain her smoke-free life.

Lesson 5: Sustaining Commitment

1. Remaining Alert

Being aware of your progress is critical for lasting success. Even after quitting, it's important to stay mindful of triggers and possible relapse scenarios.

Tip: Regularly reflect on your achievements and recall your reasons for quitting.

2. Celebrating Achievements

Acknowledging milestones can reinforce your commitment and provide motivation. Reward yourself for your smoke-free victories.

Example: Michael marked his smoke-free anniversaries with special activities, affirming his success.

Lesson 6: Adopting a Healthy Lifestyle

1. Healthy Practices

Embracing a healthy lifestyle can bolster your quitting efforts. Regular exercise, a nutritious diet, and stress management can enhance well-being and lessen the urge to smoke.

Example: Emma's active routine and healthy eating supported her smoke-free status.

2. **Mindfulness and Calmness**

Mindfulness and relaxation methods can lower stress and anxiety, common smoking triggers. These practices foster mental clarity and emotional stability.

Tip: Integrate mindfulness, meditation, or yoga into your routine to help manage stress and cravings.

The paths of Sarah, Michael, and Emma provide a map of the diverse motivations and tactics leading to a smoke-free life. Their stories affirm that with the right blend of encouragement, tools, and determination, it is indeed possible to break the chains of addiction and enjoy a healthier, non-smoking existence.

EXPERT ADVICE AND INSIGHTS

Healthcare experts are pivotal in assisting people with their journey to stop smoking. Their specialized knowledge, which is grounded in years of practice and research-backed methods, offers essential perspectives on successful quitting techniques. Let's delve into the insights provided by a range of healthcare professionals, such as physicians, mental health experts, and smoking cessation advisors.

1. **General Practitioners' Involvement**

1.1 **Assessing and Advising**

General practitioners (GPs) usually are the go-to for those looking to give up smoking. They evaluate a person's smoking past, overall health, and their determination to quit.

Main Takeaways:

- GPs tailor advice to fit each person's health profile and smoking patterns.
- They gauge how ready a person is to quit and pinpoint potential stumbling blocks.
- GPs might suggest suitable nicotine replacement therapies (NRT) or prescription options.

1.2 Support and Follow-up

GPs provide consistent support and keep an eye on a person's quitting journey. They arrange check-ins to tackle any difficulties and tweak the quitting plan as needed.

Main Takeaways:

- Regular visits are key for monitoring success and keeping up the drive to quit.
- GPs adjust quitting strategies to align with the person's reactions and needs.
- They offer encouragement and manage any side effects from quitting aids.

2. Perspectives from Psychologists

2.1 Behavioral Approaches

Psychologists are experts in behavioral therapy, which is fundamental to quitting smoking. Methods like Cognitive-Behavioral Therapy (CBT) help people to alter smoking-linked behaviors and thought patterns.

Main Takeaways:

- CBT assists in recognizing triggers and crafting coping mechanisms.
- It includes setting achievable goals and planning actionable steps.
- The therapy builds self-belief and resilience.

2.2 Tackling Psychological Addiction

Smoking is as much a mental habit as it is a physical one. Psychologists work on the emotional and psychological elements of smoking, such as stress, anxiety, and mood swings.

Main Takeaways:

- Mindfulness and relaxation techniques can lessen stress.

- Therapy can reveal deeper psychological factors that fuel smoking habits.
- Support groups and one-on-one counseling provide emotional backing.

3. Input from Smoking Cessation Specialists

3.1 Crafting Personal Quitting Schemes

Smoking cessation experts create bespoke quitting plans that cater to an individual's unique situation. These strategies often blend several methods to enhance success.

Main Takeaways:

- Specialists combine NRT, behavioral therapy, and medications.
- Custom plans take into account personal smoking habits and lifestyle choices.
- They offer comprehensive guidance for managing cravings and withdrawal.

3.2 Providing Education and Support Tools

Cessation experts inform people about the risks of smoking and the perks of quitting. They supply resources like self-help guides, apps, and support group access.

Main Takeaways:

- Educational info boosts awareness and the motivation to quit.
- Tools like quit lines and apps provide ongoing assistance.

4. The Role of Pharmacists

4.1 Overseeing Medications

Pharmacists are essential in managing stop-smoking medications. They advise on the correct use of NRT, prescriptions like varenicline (Chantix) and bupropion (Zyban), and other aids.

Main Takeaways:

- Pharmacists ensure patients know how to use quitting aids effectively.
- They inform about potential side effects and how to handle them.
- Pharmacists can suggest combining different aids for improved results.

4.2 Easy Access and Encouragement

Pharmacists are more readily available than doctors, providing quick and convenient help for those quitting smoking. They can offer immediate aid and answer queries about cessation products.

Main Takeaways:

- Easy access to pharmacists means prompt support and advice.
- They can keep up the motivation and provide follow-up support.
- Pharmacists also direct patients to further resources and experts when necessary.

LATEST FINDINGS IN SMOKING CESSATION

Keeping up with recent findings in smoking cessation is crucial to grasp the most effective techniques and new trends. Current studies highlight innovative strategies, technologies, and approaches that boost the success rates of quitting. Here, we'll look at the latest research and what it means for giving up smoking.

1. **Innovations in Nicotine Replacement Therapy (NRT)**

1.1 **Novel NRT Options**

New research has brought about fresh NRT options that are more convenient and adaptable. These include rapid-acting nicotine products and more inconspicuous methods of delivery.

Latest Discoveries:

- Quick-release nicotine gums and lozenges offer fast relief from urges.
- Nicotine mouth sprays and inhalers allow for discreet and swift nicotine intake.
- Using several NRT products at once has been linked to better quit rates.

1.2 **Tailored NRT Strategies**

Studies stress the benefits of NRT plans customized to individual smoking habits and preferences, which improve the chances of quitting.

Latest Discoveries:

- Customized NRT programs lead to better adherence and success.
- Addiction levels, triggers, and lifestyle factors influence the choice of NRT.
- Research is ongoing to perfect NRT mixes for various smoker profiles.

2. Digital Interventions and Online Tools

2.1 Apps and Online Platforms

Smoking cessation has seen a surge in the use of apps and online platforms. These digital tools offer tailored support and tracking, simplifying the quitting process.

Latest Discoveries:

- Apps allow for immediate monitoring of smoking patterns and achievements.
- Online platforms provide personalized tips, reminders, and moral support.
- Features like virtual support communities and counseling boost user involvement.

2.2 Telehealth and Online Support

The pandemic has sped up the use of online and telehealth support for smoking cessation, which has proven effective in offering continuous support and convenience.

Latest Discoveries:

- Telehealth consultations with healthcare providers are convenient and adaptable.
- Online support groups and forums foster community and shared stories.
- Virtual counseling can be just as effective as face-to-face sessions for many.

3. **Pharmaceutical Advances**

3.1 Emerging Medications

Research continues to look for new medications that more effectively target nicotine dependence, aiming to lessen cravings, ease withdrawal, and prevent relapse.

Latest Discoveries:

- New drugs are being tested that focus on brain receptors linked to addiction.
- Medications that combine anti-depressant and anti-nicotine properties are showing potential.
- Clinical trials are assessing the effectiveness and safety of these newer options.

3.2 Combined Treatments

Using multiple pharmacological treatments together has been found to increase quit success rates. Studies back the combination of different medications to address the many facets of nicotine dependence.

Latest Discoveries:

- Pairing varenicline with NRT leads to better outcomes than using each separately.
- Dual treatments tackle both the physical and mental sides of addiction.
- Research is identifying the top combination tactics for different people.

4. Psychological and Behavioral Studies

4.1 Cognitive-Behavioral Therapy (CBT)

CBT remains a key component of quitting strategies. New research keeps affirming its value and looks into integrating it with other therapies for greater impact.

Latest Discoveries:

- CBT aids in understanding and modifying smoking-linked thoughts and actions.
- Merging CBT with drug treatments results in higher quit rates.
- Online CBT programs offer accessible and cost-efficient therapy options.

4.2 Mindfulness and Coping with Stress

Mindfulness and stress management are becoming popular additions to smoking cessation efforts, with studies supporting their role in mitigating stress-related smoking triggers.

Latest Discoveries:

- Mindfulness exercises curb cravings and bolster emotional control.
- Stress management methods like deep breathing and muscle relaxation help with withdrawal.
- Combining mindfulness with established quitting programs boosts overall effectiveness.

5. Factors from Society and Surroundings

5.1 Support from One's Social Circle

It's widely recognized that having a network of support can make a big difference when trying to stop smoking. Latest research points to the significant influence that loved ones and community support play in successfully giving up smoking.

Notable Insights:

- A solid base of social support can boost both motivation and the ability to bounce back.

- Getting family and friends involved in the journey to quit smoking leads to better accountability.
- Programs and efforts at the community level create a nurturing setting that aids in the quitting process.

5.2 The Role of the Environment

Studies are delving into how environmental elements, like rules at the workplace and bans on smoking in public, affect how many people stop smoking.

Notable Insights:

- Policies that make workplaces free from smoke help nudge workers to stop smoking and bring down the number of smokers overall.
- Bans on smoking in public places lead to fewer people smoking and less exposure to secondhand smoke.
- Establishing a smoke-free zone at home can be a big help for those trying to quit.

YOUR NEW BEGINNING

Kicking the smoking habit marks a tremendous stride in safeguarding your health and enhancing your overall quality of life. As you step into this fresh start, it's vital to pause and ponder over the path you've traveled. Reflecting isn't just about reinforcing your determination; it's about valuing every step forward and the obstacles you've conquered.

1. **Saluting Your Hard Work**

1.1 **Cheering Every Triumph**

The road to quitting smoking is paved with numerous small triumphs. Every cigarette you've turned down, each craving you've weathered, and every day you've remained smoke-free counts as a win worth celebrating.

Key Points:

- Applaud each and every milestone, no matter the size.

- Maintain a diary to track your successes and mull over your advancements.
- Give yourself credit for the grit and resolve you've shown in quitting.

1.2 Looking Back at Triumphs Over Trials

Grasping the hurdles you've surmounted can offer profound insights and fortitude. Reflecting on these instances highlights your tenacity and your capacity to tackle tough times.

Key Points:

- Pinpoint the toughest moments and how you conquered them.
- Think about the tactics that served you well during those challenges.
- Contemplate what these experiences have taught you about your endurance and adaptability.

2. **Grasping the Gains**

2.1 Health Enhancements

Mulling over the health perks you've noticed since quitting can bolster your pledge to stay smoke-free. Better breathing, a surge in vitality, and overall health improvement are just a few of the positive shifts you might notice.

Key Points:

- Observe physical improvements like easier breathing, healthier skin, and more energy.
- Consider the positive effects quitting has had on your mental well-being and mood.
- Be grateful for the long-term health benefits, including a lower risk of heart disease and cancer.

2.2 Self-Improvement

Quitting smoking is as much about personal transformation as it is about health. Reflecting on this evolution can help you see how much you've changed and the new strengths you've cultivated.

Key Points:

- Think about the impact quitting has had on your self-worth and confidence.
- Look at the new skills and habits you've picked up, such as managing stress and adopting healthier coping mechanisms.

- Acknowledge how your smoke-free life has positively influenced your relationships and social life.

3. **Drawing Lessons from Setbacks**

3.1 **Examining Relapse Triggers**

If relapses were part of your journey, looking back on these instances can be incredibly instructive. Understanding what led to a relapse arms you with knowledge to handle similar situations better in the future.

Key Points:

- Identify the triggers and risky scenarios that led to slip-ups.
- Reflect on your emotional and mental state at those times.
- Plan out ways to sidestep or manage these triggers going forward.

3.2 **Crafting a Resilience Strategy**

Based on your past experiences, devising a resilience strategy can solidify your commitment and ready you for future hurdles.

Key Points:

- Compile a list of coping mechanisms for stress and cravings.
- Prepare for social settings and environments where smoking might be tempting.
- Make sure you have a support system to lean on when you need a boost.

Taking time to reflect is a crucial component of your new start. It helps you acknowledge how far you've come, understand the advantages of quitting, and learn from any setbacks or relapses. These reflections fortify your dedication to a life without smoke and set you up for ongoing success.

Welcoming Your Smoke-Free Life

Here comes the excitement and the moment we all had been waiting for.

Welcoming your smoke-free life means gazing ahead with hope and enthusiasm. It's about embracing the new doors that open when you lead a healthier, smoke-free existence. This segment delves into how to cherish your fresh start and maximize your smoke-free life.

1. **Crafting New Ambitions**

1.1 **Health and Fitness Ambitions**

Now that you've left smoking behind, you can channel your energy into new health and fitness ambitions. Whether you're eyeing a marathon, thinking about joining a gym, or just wanting to be more active, these goals can drive you and bring a sense of fulfillment.

Key Points:

- Aim for SMART (specific, measurable, attainable, relevant, and time-bound) goals.
- Make regular exercise a part of your life to keep up your health and spirits.
- Try out new physical activities and pastimes that you find enjoyable.

1.2 **Personal and Career Ambitions**

Quitting smoking can unleash a newfound sense of empowerment and assurance, which you can channel into personal and career ambitions. Whether it's climbing the career ladder, mastering a new skill, or chasing a dream, now's the time to set and chase new dreams.

Key Points:

- Pin down areas in your life you'd like to enhance or expand.
- Set goals that are both realistic and stimulating, aligning with what you value and are passionate about.
- Celebrate your triumphs and let them fuel your drive for further achievements.

2. **Adopting Wholesome Routines**

2.1 **Nutrition and Eating Habits**

A well-rounded diet is key to keeping up your health and energy. Concentrate on integrating nourishing foods into your diet and steering clear of unhealthy habits.

Key Points:

- Organize meals rich in fruits, veggies, lean proteins, and whole grains.
- Stay well-hydrated and moderate your caffeine and sugar intake.
- Think about getting tailored dietary advice from a nutritionist.

2.2 Managing Stress

Mastering stress management is vital for sustaining your smoke-free lifestyle. Cultivate healthy habits and techniques to handle stress without falling back on smoking.

Key Points:

- Embrace mindfulness and relaxation methods like deep breathing, meditation, and yoga.
- Engage in regular physical activity to alleviate stress and elevate your mood.
- Find pastimes and activities that you enjoy and that help you unwind.

3. **Bolstering Your Circle of Support**

3.1 Connecting with Kin and Friends

Fostering robust connections with friends and family can give you the emotional support and encouragement you need. Share your story and revel in your achievements with those close to you.

Key Points:

- Talk openly with your dear ones about your experiences and emotions.
- Spend meaningful time with friends and family to strengthen your connections.
- Rely on your support network when times get tough.

3.2 Engaging with Support Groups

Linking up with others who've quit smoking or are on the same path can offer extra support and drive. Join support groups or online communities to exchange stories and tips.

Key Points:

- Get involved in local or online support groups to keep in touch with those who get your struggles.
- Offer your insights and lend a hand to others on their quitting journey.
- Use these connections to stay inspired and accountable.

WORDS TO KEEP YOU GOING

Quitting smoking is an impressive feat that speaks to your resolve, persistence, and resilience. As you press on with your smoke-free path, it's key to keep the motivation high and recall the reasons you quit. Here are some final words of encouragement to keep you steadfast and uplifted.

1. **Applauding Your Victories**

1.1 Acknowledge Your Success

Quitting smoking is a noteworthy achievement that warrants celebration. Rejoice in your success and take pride in how far you've come.

Key Points:

- Reflect on your journey and the effort and determination it demanded to quit.
- Mark your milestones and victories with treats that delight you.
- Spread the word about your accomplishment and be a beacon for others.

1.2 Be an Inspiration

Your story of success can motivate others trying to break free from smoking. Share your experiences and offer a helping hand and words of encouragement to those still battling the habit.

Key Points:

- Be a beacon of hope and encouragement for others aiming to quit.
- Share what worked for you to help others carve their own path to success.
- Celebrate the strides of those you've inspired and continue to back them up.

2. Maintaining Dedication

2.1 Keeping Your Motivation in Sight

Constantly remind yourself of the compelling reasons that led you to give up smoking. Holding on to these motivations can anchor your dedication and keep you focused on a future without smoke.

Essential Thoughts:

- Jot down your quitting motives and place them where you'll frequently see them.
- Contemplate the positive changes in your life and health since you stopped smoking.
- Draw on these motivations to bolster your resolve when times get tough.

2.2 Readying for Hurdles

You've come a long way, but it's crucial to stay ready for any obstacles ahead. Keep a keen eye out and have strategies ready to tackle any triggers or cravings that may arise.

Essential Thoughts:

- Pinpoint triggers that could tempt you and plan ways to counter them.
- Cultivate healthy habits and routines that reinforce your commitment to being smoke-free.
- Lean on your support circle for extra motivation and guidance when needed.

3. Adopting an Optimistic Attitude

3.1 Accentuating the Positive

Adopting an optimistic attitude is key to your smoke-free journey. Concentrate on the gains you've made since quitting and the positive shifts in your life.

Essential Thoughts:

- Celebrate your health improvements, increased vitality, and overall betterment.
- Relish the newfound autonomy and control you've reclaimed by stopping smoking.
- Maintain an upbeat perspective and look forward to a more wholesome future.

3.2 Keeping the Drive Alive

Fuel your motivation by setting fresh objectives and embracing new challenges. Continuously seek personal development and progress.

Essential Thoughts:

- Establish new health and fitness objectives to stay driven and active.
- Engage in hobbies and pursuits that spark joy and a sense of achievement, ensuring a rich and fulfilling smoke-free life.

HELPFUL RESOURCES AND WORKSHEETS
Goal-Setting Blueprints

Crafting well-defined goals is fundamental to successfully giving up smoking. These goals serve as your compass, providing both motivation and direction. Goal-setting blueprints are instrumental in organizing your aims, making them more reachable and measurable. We'll delve into how to devise and apply effective goal-setting blueprints as you embark on your smoke-free journey.

1. The Significance of Goal Setting

1.1 The Role of Goals

Goals are pivotal in mapping out your path to quitting smoking. They turn your vague wish to stop into specific, quantifiable milestones.

Key Takeaways:

- Goals fuel your drive and give you a clear purpose.
- They break the quitting journey into smaller, achievable chunks.
- Reaching these goals boosts your self-assurance and solidifies your dedication.

1.2 SMART Goals Framework

Adopting the **SMART** criteria ensures your goals are well-defined and within reach.

2. Crafting Your Goal-Setting Blueprint

2.1 Elements of a Goal-Setting Blueprint

A robust goal-setting blueprint comprises essential elements that steer you toward setting and hitting your targets.

Key Takeaways:

- ✓ **Goal Declaration:** State your objective clearly.

- ✓ **Justification**: Clarify why this goal matters to you.
- ✓ **Action Steps**: Chart the course of actions to reach your goal.
- ✓ **Schedule**: Assign deadlines for each action and the goal as a whole.
- ✓ **Monitoring Progress**: Make space for tracking your advancements and tweaking your plan when necessary.

2.2 Blueprint Examples

Seeing examples of structured goal-setting blueprints can spark ideas and direction as you craft your personalized version.

Example 1:

Goal Declaration: Cut down from 10 to 5 cigarettes daily within a month.

Justification: Lessening my smoking will benefit my health and ease the transition to quitting completely.

Action Steps:

- Week 1: Limit to 8 cigarettes daily.
- Week 2: Cut back to 6 cigarettes daily.
- Week 3: Maintain at 5 cigarettes daily.

Schedule: Start: June 1, Finish: June 30.

Monitoring Progress: Keep a daily tally of cigarettes smoked.

Example 2:

Goal Declaration: Completely stop smoking by year's end.

Justification: Quitting smoking will greatly enhance my health and life quality.

Action Steps:

- Months 1-3: Halve cigarette use.
- Months 4-6: Switch to nicotine replacement therapy.
- Months 7-9: Taper off nicotine replacement use.
- Months 10-12: Stop using nicotine products entirely.

Schedule: Start: January 1, Finish: December 31.

Monitoring Progress: Monthly check-ins with a healthcare professional.

3. Implementing Your Goal-Setting Blueprint

3.1 Putting Your Blueprint to Work

With your goal-setting blueprint ready, it's time for action. Regular check-ins and adaptability are crucial to remain on course.

Key Takeaways:

- Regularly revisit your goals to track your headway.
- Modify your plan as needed, considering your progress and any obstacles faced.
- Keep your resolve by recalling the benefits of quitting smoking.

3.2 Keeping the Drive Alive

Staying driven on your quit-smoking path can be tough. Goal-setting blueprints can help maintain focus and enthusiasm.

Key Takeaways:

- Celebrate every little victory and milestone.

- Envision the long-term gains of reaching your goals.
- Lean on support from loved ones and support networks.

Goal-setting blueprints are potent aids in your quest to quit smoking. They lend structure and clarity, translating your quitting aspiration into actionable steps and tangible results. Regular reviews and updates to your blueprint can keep you inspired and on the right path, committed to your smoke-free future.

PROGRESS MONITORING CHARTS

Keeping tabs on your progress is vital in your cessation of smoking. Progress monitoring charts offer a structured way to oversee your achievements, discern patterns, and fine-tune your tactics accordingly. We'll examine the value of progress tracking, the elements of successful progress monitoring charts, and their effective use.

1. **The Value of Progress Tracking**

1.1 **Success Assessment**

Tracking your progress sheds light on your journey's distance and proximity to your goals. It's a source of fulfillment and a motivational booster.

Key Takeaways:

- Progress tracking visualizes your path and accomplishments.
- It supplies data that can spur you to persist.
- Consistent checks can spotlight areas for improvement.

1.2 Detecting Patterns and Triggers

Keeping track helps pinpoint patterns and triggers impacting your quit-smoking journey. Comprehending these aids in formulating strategies to conquer them.

Key Takeaways:

- Spot times or scenarios when cravings hit hardest.
- Detect emotional or situational prompts to smoke.
- Use these insights to sidestep triggers or devise coping methods.

2. **Developing Your Progress Monitoring Chart**

2.1 Progress Monitoring Chart Elements

A comprehensive progress monitoring chart includes various elements that collectively aid in a thorough tracking of your quitting process.

Key Takeaways:

- **Date**: Log the date for daily progress records.
- **Cigarette Count**: Keep a daily tally of cigarettes consumed.
- **Craving Notes**: Record the intensity and regularity of cravings.
- **Trigger Identification**: Note any triggers faced throughout the day.
- **Applied Strategies**: Jot down the techniques employed to resist smoking.
- **Observations**: Add any further remarks or findings.

2.2 Chart Examples

Examples of progress monitoring charts can guide you in creating a chart that suits your specific needs.

Example 1:

Date: June 1

Cigarette Count: 8

Craving Notes: Strong in the morning, moderate by night.

Trigger Identification: Work stress, socializing.

Applied Strategies: Breathing exercises, chewing gum.

Observations: Felt more in command despite stress.

Example 2:

Date: June 2

Cigarette Count: 7

Craving Notes: Steady moderate cravings.

Trigger Identification: Coffee breaks, post-meal times.

Applied Strategies: Walks during breaks, sipping water.

Observations: Cut down on smoking, feeling upbeat.

3. <u>Utilizing Your Progress Monitoring Chart</u>

3.1 **Regular Tracking**

For your progress monitoring to be effective, consistency is essential. Fill in your chart daily for an accurate reflection of your journey.

Key Takeaways:

- Pick a set time each day for your chart update.
- Record honestly and in detail for true insights.
- Regularly review your chart to observe trends and implement changes.

3.2 Interpreting Data

Making it a habit to examine your tracking data can reveal crucial insights into your process of quitting. Leverage this data to tweak your methods and keep yourself aligned with your goals.

Main Takeaways:

- Search for recurring themes in your cravings and what sets them off.
- Discover which techniques work best for you personally.
- Revise your plan of action based on the discoveries and progress you make.

TRIGGER RECOGNITION WORKSHEETS

Grasping and managing what triggers your smoking is a fundamental aspect of quitting. Triggers are those circumstances, emotional states, or settings that provoke a desire to smoke. Trigger recognition worksheets are designed to help you acknowledge these triggers and formulate plans to cope with them. This section delves into why it's important to identify triggers, what makes worksheets effective, and how they can aid your quitting efforts.

1. Why Identifying Triggers Matters

1.1 Detecting Recurring Patterns

Spotting your triggers is key to understanding the recurring patterns and contexts that lead to your smoking urges. Being aware is essential for coming up with successful coping mechanisms.

Main Takeaways:

- Detecting triggers enables you to steer clear of or handle risky scenarios.
- Grasping these patterns lets you anticipate and ready yourself for cravings.
- Realizing what your triggers are is a critical step towards breaking free from smoking.

1.2 Minimizing the Chance of Relapse

Being knowledgeable about your triggers and the ways to manage them lowers the chances of falling back into smoking. It arms you with the necessary tools to stay smoke-free.

Main Takeaways:

- Managing triggers well is crucial to fend off relapses.
- Crafting coping strategies for your triggers builds up your resilience.
- Limiting your exposure to triggers helps solidify your resolve to quit.

2. Crafting Effective Trigger Recognition Worksheets

2.1 What Goes into a Trigger Recognition Worksheet

A well-constructed trigger recognition worksheet includes several elements that assist in identifying and dealing with your smoking triggers.

Main Takeaways:

- ✓ **Trigger Detailing**: Pinpoint and depict the exact trigger.

- ✓ **Context**: Record the circumstances or environment where the trigger appears.
- ✓ **Emotional Response**: Jot down the emotions you feel when encountering the trigger.
- ✓ **Urge Strength**: Evaluate the strength of the urge on a scale (for instance, from 1 to 10).
- ✓ **Management Techniques**: Enumerate the techniques you employed or intend to employ to deal with the trigger.
- ✓ **Result**: Note down the effectiveness of your management technique (for example, Was it successful? Did you give in to smoking?).

2.2 Samples of Trigger Identification Worksheets

Access to samples of structured trigger identification worksheets can serve as a template for devising your tailored worksheets.

Example A:

Trigger Detailing: Morning cup of coffee.

Context: Sipping coffee solo at the kitchen counter.

Emotional Response: Peaceful yet a routine compulsion to smoke.

Urge Strength: 7 out of 10, so let's say urge is still high.

Management Techniques: Sipping water right after coffee, munching on gum.

Result: Successfully refrained from smoking, urge dropped to 3.

Example B:

Trigger Detailing: Workplace stress.

Context: Getting a stern email from the supervisor.

Emotional Response: Nervousness, irritation.

Urge Strength: 9

Management Techniques: Stepping out for a brief walk, practicing deep breathing.

Result: Managed to postpone the urge, stayed smoke-free, urge reduced to 5.

3. Implementing Trigger Identification Worksheets

3.1 Keeping Your Worksheet Up-to-Date

Steady use of trigger identification worksheets is crucial. Keeping your worksheet current ensures you remain conscious of your triggers and can fine-tune your management techniques.

Main Takeaways:

- Fill in the worksheet right after a craving hit to ensure the details are fresh and precise.
- Go over your worksheet on a weekly basis to spot trends and gauge the success of your methods.
- Modify your management techniques drawing on insights from your worksheet.

3.2 Crafting a Tailored Strategy

Leverage the knowledge from your trigger identification worksheets to establish a customized strategy for confronting triggers. Your strategy should be adaptable and grow with your accumulating experience.

Main Takeaways:

- Sort your triggers by their intensity and how often they occur.
- Formulate targeted management techniques for each trigger that's a top concern.
- Weave these techniques into your routine to ready yourself for and navigate through cravings effectively.

COMMONLY ASKED QUESTIONS ABOUT QUITTING SMOKING

Quitting smoking is a significant step towards better health and a longer life. It's okay to have questions and concerns as you embark on this journey. Here are answers to some of the most commonly asked questions about quitting smoking, which can provide clarity, guidance, and encouragement.

1. Why Should I Quit Smoking?

Health Benefits

Quitting smoking dramatically reduces your risk of numerous health problems, including heart disease, stroke, lung disease, and various types of cancer. Within weeks of quitting, you'll experience improved lung function and circulation, and within a year, your risk of coronary heart disease is cut in half.

Financial Savings

Smoking is an expensive habit. The cost of cigarettes adds up over time, and quitting can save you a significant amount of money. These savings can be redirected towards healthier activities and investments.

Quality of Life

Non-smokers generally have a better quality of life. They enjoy increased energy levels, better taste and smell, improved skin health, and reduced coughing and shortness of breath. Quitting smoking also positively impacts the health of those around you, especially children and non-smoking adults.

2. How Can I Prepare to Quit Smoking?

Set a Quit Date

Choosing a specific date to quit can help you mentally prepare for the change. Select a day within the next two weeks to give yourself enough time to get ready without losing motivation.

Identify Triggers

Recognize the situations, emotions, and habits that trigger your urge to smoke. Common triggers include stress, social gatherings, drinking alcohol, and specific times of the day.

Develop a Plan

Create a detailed quit plan that includes your quit date, strategies to handle triggers, and a list of support resources. This plan will serve as a roadmap to guide you through the quitting process.

3. What Are Some Effective Strategies for Quitting Smoking?

Cold Turkey

Quitting abruptly, or "cold turkey," is a method where you stop smoking completely on your quit date without the use of any aids. While challenging, many people succeed with this method.

Gradual Reduction

Slowly reducing the number of cigarettes, you smoke each day until you quit completely can help ease the transition and reduce withdrawal symptoms.

Nicotine Replacement Therapy (NRT)

NRT provides low doses of nicotine without the harmful chemicals found in cigarettes. Options include nicotine patches, gum, lozenges, inhalers, and nasal sprays.

Prescription Medications

Behavioral Therapy

Behavioral therapies, including cognitive-behavioral therapy (CBT), hypnotherapy, and mindfulness techniques, can help you develop strategies to cope with cravings and triggers.

4. What Are the Withdrawal Symptoms and How Can I Manage Them?

Common Withdrawal Symptoms

When you quit smoking, you may experience withdrawal symptoms such as irritability, anxiety, difficulty concentrating, increased appetite, and strong cravings for nicotine.

Managing Withdrawal Symptoms

- Stay Hydrated: Drinking plenty of water can help flush nicotine out of your system.
- Stay Active
- Healthy Diet: Eating a balanced diet can help manage weight gain and keep your energy levels stable.
- Support Network: Rely on friends, family, support groups, or counseling to help you through tough times.

5. How to effectively manage cravings and triggers?

Distraction Techniques

Engage in activities that keep your mind and hands busy, such as hobbies, exercise, or spending time with friends and family.

Substitute Behaviors

Find healthier alternatives to smoking, such as chewing gum, eating healthy snacks, or practicing deep breathing exercises.

Avoiding Triggers

Avoid and identify situations that trigger the urge to smoke. This might mean temporarily avoiding certain social situations or places where you used to smoke.

6. What if I Relapse?

Understanding Relapse

Relapsing is common and doesn't mean you've failed. It's an opportunity to learn more about your triggers and develop stronger strategies for the future.

Getting Back on Track

If you relapse, don't be too hard on yourself. Analyze what led to the relapse, and adjust your quit plan to address those factors. Set a new quit date and keep trying.

Seeking Support

Reach out to your support network or a healthcare professional for guidance and encouragement. They can help you identify what went wrong and how to prevent it from happening again.

7. What Resources Are Available to Help Me Quit Smoking?

Quitline

Many countries offer free Quitline that provide support and resources for people trying to quit smoking. These services can offer personalized advice and counseling.

Support Groups

Joining a support group, either in person or online, can provide you with encouragement, tips, and accountability from others who are also quitting smoking.

Healthcare Providers

Consulting with your doctor or a smoking cessation specialist can provide you with personalized advice and access to medications and therapies that can help you quit.

8. How Can I Maintain My Smoke-Free Status?

Stay Vigilant

Even after you've quit, it's important to remain aware of your triggers and avoid situations that might tempt you to smoke.

Celebrate Milestones

Celebrate your progress and milestones, no matter how small. Recognizing your achievements can help keep you motivated.

Adopt a Healthy Lifestyle

Maintaining a healthy lifestyle, including regular exercise, a balanced diet, and stress management techniques, can help you stay smoke-free.

Continuous Learning

Continue educating yourself about the benefits of quitting and the risks of smoking. Knowledge can reinforce your commitment to a smoke-free life.

Quit smoking the easy way

A HAPPY NON-SMOKER

CONGRATULATIONS.

www.ingramcontent.com/pod-product-compliance
Lightning Source LLC
Chambersburg PA
CBHW071913210526
45479CB00002B/404